THE 28-DAY PEGAN DIET

More than 120 Easy Recipes for Healthy Weight Loss

Isabel Minunni

with Aimee McNew, MNT, CNTP

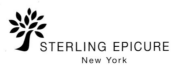

STERLING EPICURE
New York

introduction

THOUGH THIS BOOK includes a plan for eating pegan for 28 days, you shouldn't think of it as a fad, cleanse or any other short-term solution. Instead, think of it as the best way for you to reset your body and jump into the exciting world of pegan eating. According to its creator Dr. Mark Hyman, pegan, or paleo-vegan, is a diet you should embrace for the rest of your life. This extremely flexible plan combines the best parts of vegan and paleo diets, helping people live healthier, more satisfying lives. So what are you waiting for? It's time to start eating pegan and start feeling good, inside and out.

contents

4
what is the pegan diet?

15
why pegan is one of the best diets

24
pegan cheat sheet

25
the pegan pantry

26
28-day pegan meal plan

32
substitutions

33
conversions

35 breakfast	**123** sides
65 snacks & starters	**151** mains
95 soups & salads	**189** dessert

219
references

220
index

What Is the Pegan Diet?

Part paleo, part vegan, the pegan diet isn't simply a combination of these two diametrically opposed dietary programs.

AT FIRST GLANCE, it seems the paleo diet, which involves eating high-quality meats, eggs and animal fats, and the vegan diet, which avoids anything remotely derived from animals, are incompatible.

The term, pegan, was coined by Dr. Mark Hyman in a blog post on his website that was published November 7, 2014. The director of the Cleveland Clinic Center for Functional Medicine claimed that his inspiration for combining aspects of paleo with the vegan diet came from research that demonstrates both can have health-promoting qualities.

Both paleo and vegan are known for promoting natural weight loss, lowering cholesterol and reversing diabetes. But with both approaches so fundamentally different, which one is the right one? Hyman suggests you can be both.

Hyman said in his original pegan blog post: "I vote for being a pegan or paleo-vegan, which is what I have chosen for myself and recommend for most of my patients. Keep in mind that most of us need to personalize the approach depending on our health conditions, preferences and needs."

PRINCIPLES OF THE PEGAN DIET

When people hear that the pegan diet is part paleo and part vegan, they often assume it simply combines what the two diets have in common. Yet the only overlapping foods between the two are fruits, vegetables, nuts and seeds—a hunger-inducing diet, for sure.

Instead, Hyman says the overarching principle in common between paleo and being a healthy vegan is the primary focus on "real, whole, fresh food that is sustainably raised."

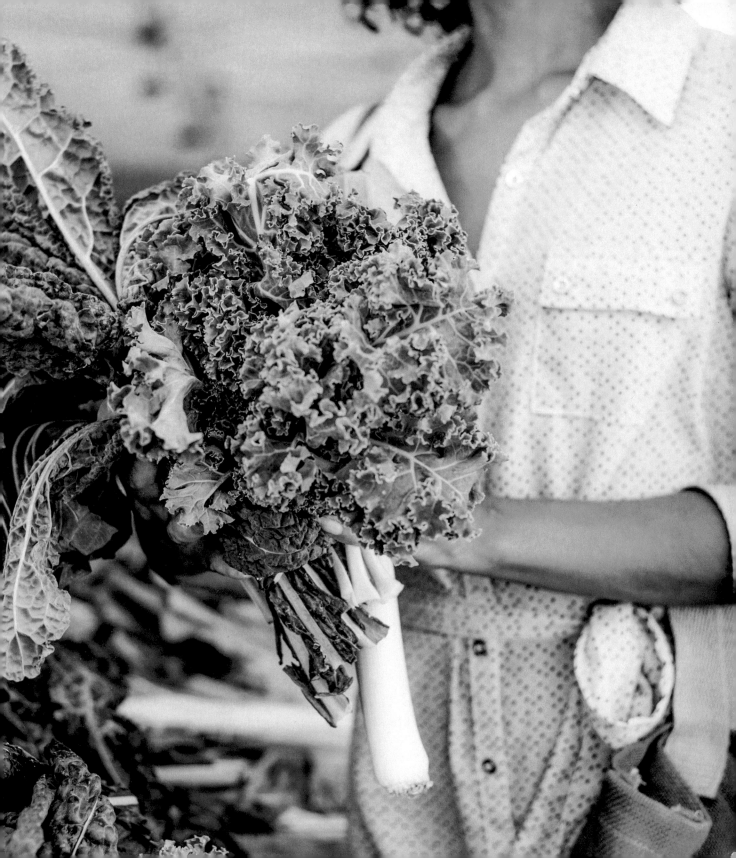

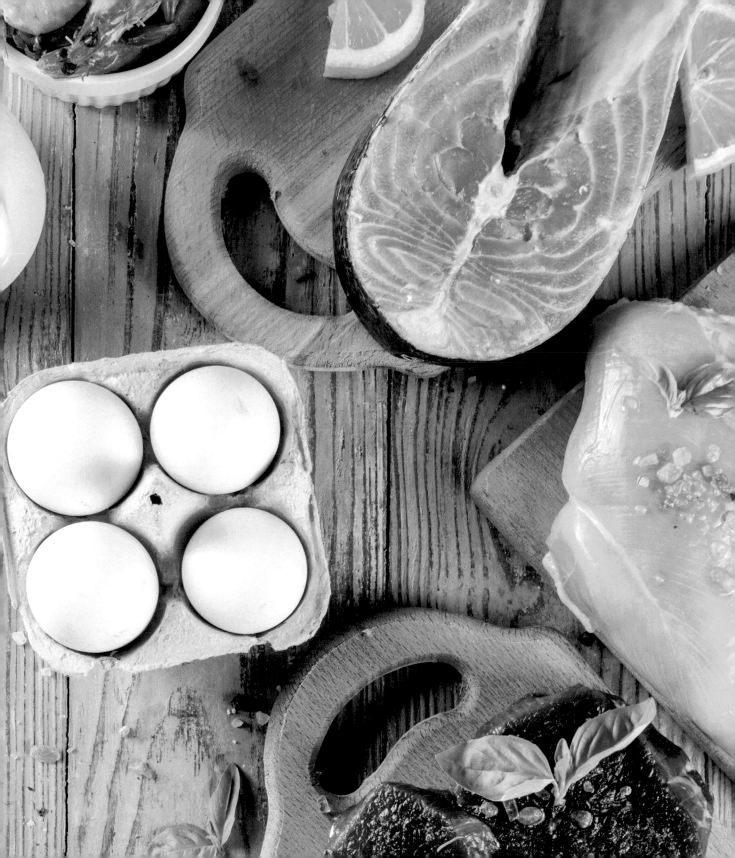

The principles that both diets agree on, and that Hyman outlined in his original pegan post, are:

- Plenty of vegetables and fruits
- Low glycemic load (very low sugar, flour and refined carbohydrates)
- Organic, local and fresh foods that are low in pesticides, antibiotics, hormones and GMOs
- Adequate protein intake
- Foods free from chemicals, additives, dyes, preservatives, MSG and artificial sweeteners
- Higher intake of good-quality omega-3 fats

For the purposes of pairing paleo with vegan, it is additionally important to focus on sustainably raised animal products, such as those that are wild-caught, free-range and grass-fed. Fish should be those that are low in mercury and toxins, such as sardines, herring, mackerel and anchovies. Tuna, swordfish and Chilean sea bass should be avoided because of their higher mercury levels.

While most paleo and vegan eaters can come together on the previous recommendations, some aspects of the pegan diet will confuse or frustrate eaters from both camps. In these cases, Hyman backs up his recommendations with research.

WHAT YOU CAN EAT ON A PEGAN DIET

A pegan diet is far from calorie-restricted and focuses on nourishing the body. It is not meant to be a starvation diet and offers a wide range of personalization to address individual needs.

Pegan eaters can expect to consume the following:

FISH

Seafood is rich in omega-3 fatty acids that fight inflammation in the body and promote overall wellness. The modern American diet is overloaded in omega-6 fats, typically from nuts, seeds and vegetable oils. Increasing seafood intake is essential to balance the ratio.

Mercury in fish is a serious concern, however. All seafood does not offer the same benefits. For pegan purposes, choose low-mercury fish like salmon, mackerel, sardines and anchovies. Always ensure fish is wild-caught and not farm-raised.

Dr. Hyman notes omega-3 fats are still essential, so if you don't eat seafood, supplement with high-quality EPA and DHA from fish oil. If you don't eat fish for moral reasons, you can still get the omega-3s you need from algae.

EGGS

An excellent source of folate, protein and even 10 percent daily value of vitamin D, eggs are a nutrient-packed food. Cholesterol was long blamed as the cause of heart disease, but modern research proves otherwise. Eggs are a great food to eat on a pegan diet for those who can digest them. Some with autoimmune issues or egg allergies will want to avoid eggs.

MEAT

While meat is certainly allowed on a pegan diet, not all meat is healthy or compatible. Beef from feedlot operations is pumped full of hormones, antibiotics and other chemicals that lead to overall reduced quality of food products.

When choosing meat on a pegan diet, it should be sourced from farms where meat is treated ethically, primarily grass-fed and allowed to roam free. Chickens should be pastured. Eating sustainably sourced meat isn't only about the health benefits either. It also supports better environmental health.

Hyman notes that some research shows meat increases the risk of heart disease and death rates, while other research shows the opposite. Hyman believes the overall evidence leads to meat not being linked to death or heart attacks. Perhaps the most important shift in thinking regarding the paleo diet versus the pegan diet is that on the pegan plan, meat should be viewed as a side dish as opposed to the main course.

VEGETABLES AND FRUIT

Both paleo and vegan diets encourage plenty of fresh, organic and, when possible, locally sourced produce. While paleo tends to encourage lower glycemic fruits like berries, technically any fruits and veggies are game for pegan. If you have diabetes, consider sticking to low-glycemic options and ensuring vegetable intake is higher.

Dried fruits are often considered fruit, but for pegan, paleo or vegan, they are a gray area since they are substantially higher in sugar. Consume them rarely and in extreme moderation, first opting for fresh fruits instead.

Many dieters also want to know about juicing, but since this removes the fiber and roughage from produce, it's best to eat fruits and vegetables whole or in smoothies and not juiced. Juicing can also produce a high-sugar product, even though it's fresh.

Processed fruit and vegetable juice contains preservatives and other ingredients that make it a far cry from fresh produce, so avoid these on a pegan diet.

Overall, Hyman says 75 percent of the plate for pegan meals should be low-glycemic fruits and vegetables.

NUTS AND SEEDS

Nuts and seeds are a staple of many vegan diets and are commonly found on paleo diets as well.

Ranging from minerals to fiber to protein, nuts and seeds have many nutritional benefits.

One downside, though, is that they contain phytates and antinutrients, which can make them difficult to digest for some, especially when eaten in large quantities. Soaking or sprouting nuts and seeds can help to improve digestibility and nutrient content.

Nuts and seeds also contain more omega-6 fatty acids than omega-3s, so it's important to eat them in moderation and in balance with omega-3 fatty foods.

They're allowed on a pegan diet, but should be a small portion or side and should take a back seat to vegetables and fruits.

GRAINS

While paleo is a grain-free diet, the pegan diet allows moderate amounts of certain grains. It does, however, strictly avoid gluten. According to Hyman, gluten "creates inflammation, autoimmunity and digestive disorders" for millions of Americans. He says gluten is even linked with obesity.

Pegan allows certain grains but always recommends small portions of ½ cup or less per meal. Low-glycemic grains are preferred, such as black rice and quinoa.

Hyman recommends a grain-free pegan diet for those who have diabetes and autoimmune disease.

BEANS AND LEGUMES

A primary source of protein and fiber for vegan diets, beans are completely avoided on paleo diets because they contain antinutrients that make them hard to digest and interfere with nutrient absorption. So which view is right?

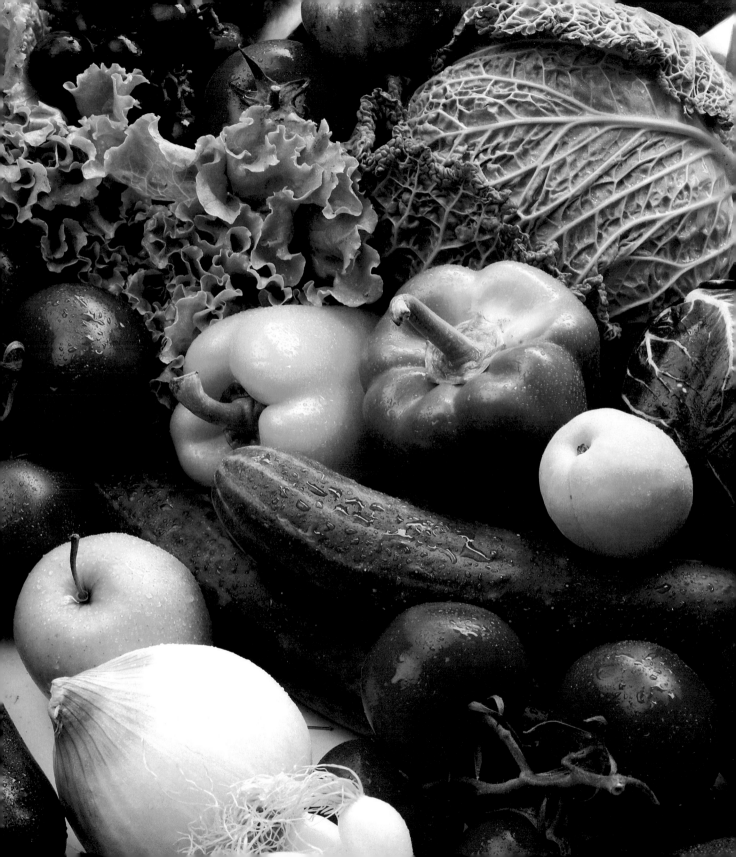

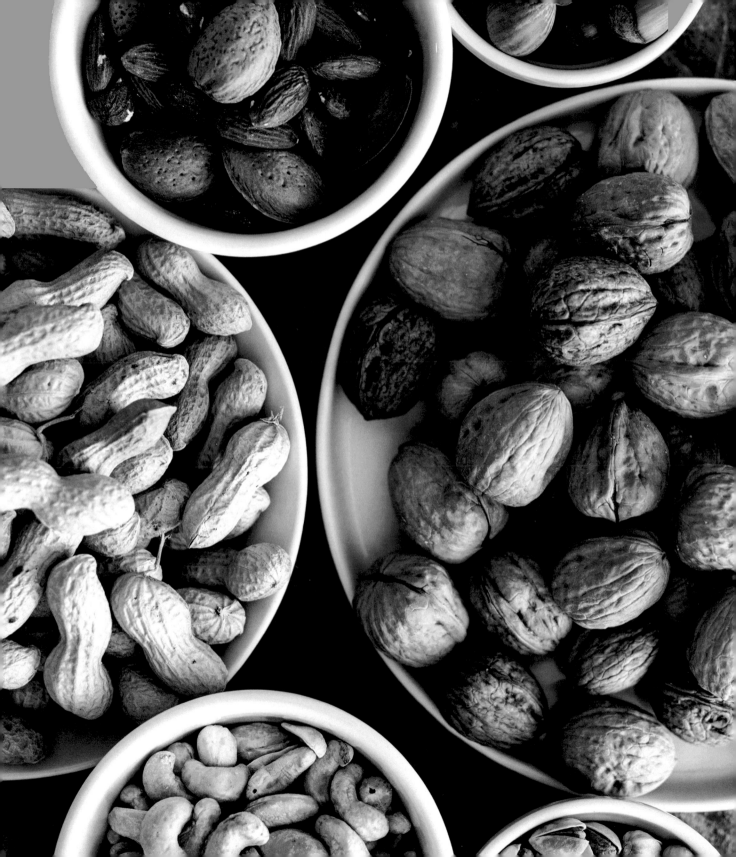

Hyman notes that beans are problematic for those who get digestive symptoms when they eat them or for diabetics, for whom beans can spike blood sugar levels. He recommends up to 1 cup of beans per day for those who are not sensitive or diabetic.

FATS AND OILS
Hyman stresses the importance of the right types of fats on a pegan diet. In addition to seafood and grass-fed meats, he encourages avoiding vegetable oils like canola, corn, soybean and sunflower, opting instead for coconut oil, olive oil, avocado oil and saturated fats from grass-fed animal products, like ghee and butter.

SUPPLEMENTS
While it's always wise to check with your doctor before starting any supplements, Hyman notes that two nutrients might be especially important for supplementation on a pegan diet. These include vitamin D3 and vitamin B12 (for those who eat mostly vegan).

D3 is not found in an abundance of food sources, and without regular sunscreen-free exposure to the sun, it is difficult to obtain enough vitamin D from food alone. Vitamin D is needed for a healthy brain, normal immunity and thyroid health.

B12 is found in plenty of animal products, but those who don't eat meat or eat it infrequently might be low on this vital nutrient that supports the nervous system, muscular health and healthy red blood cells.

DAIRY ON A PEGAN DIET?
Neither the paleo diet nor vegan diets use dairy products. Hyman notes that most adults cannot tolerate cow's milk and that it can contribute to obesity, diabetes, heart disease, cancer and more.

In his original blog post for the pegan diet, Hyman counsels avoiding dairy from cows but recommends trying sheep or goat milk products for an occasional treat. These products should always be organic.

For those who cannot digest even these forms of milk, it's easy to swap them for plant-based milk, like almond, cashew, hemp, coconut or oat milk. In most recipes these kinds of milk swap one-for-one, although the different thickness or taste may alter the recipe slightly.

HOW PEGAN IS DIFFERENT FROM OTHER POPULAR DIETS
The pegan diet is one of the newer dietary trends to rise in popularity. Here's how it stacks up against other recently popular food plans.

PALEO
The paleo diet focuses on high-quality animal products like meat, seafood and eggs, along with fats, vegetables, fruits, nuts and seeds. Paleo avoids all grains, dairy, legumes, refined sugar and processed foods. Since pegan is partly derived from paleo, there are many similarities, with key differences being that pegan allows certain grains, beans, legumes and limited dairy.

VEGAN
The other component that inspired the creation of pegan, a vegan diet avoids all animal products or anything that has a mother. It focuses on plant-based food products entirely, even avoiding anything made with animal-based derivatives. The pegan diet aims to choose sustainably

sourced food that is mindful of the environment, much like veganism, but does allow meat and other animal products in moderation. Both vegan and pegan stress the importance of vegetables and fruit.

VEGETARIAN

Less strict than vegan, there are several variations of vegetarianism. Some allow fish and eggs, whereas others allow dairy. Vegetarian eaters may find a lot in common with pegan eating principles, including the meat and animal products in moderate amounts.

KETO

An extreme high-fat, low-carb diet, keto focuses on mostly fat, moderate protein and very little carbohydrates. By nature, keto is lower in vegetables and fruit because both contain carbs, and is significantly higher in fats and meat than the pegan diet. While it is possible to be paleo-keto, it is much harder to follow a pegan diet while eating keto because it would be difficult to make the plate 75 percent vegetables and fruit.

DASH

The DASH diet stands for Dietary Approaches to Stop Hypertension and is often used when cholesterol is high, heart disease risk is increased or diabetes is present. DASH focuses on significantly lower sodium levels than the standard American diet and includes plenty of vegetables, fruits, whole grains and low-fat dairy. DASH encourages up to six to eight servings of grains daily. It also stresses only lean meats, poultry and fish, and limiting fats and oils to two servings per day. DASH and pegan stand opposite on some important factors. Pegan encourages grains in moderation, while DASH pushes grains as the primary food group. DASH counts sodium and urges low-fat dairy, while pegan disregards sodium as a factor when processed foods are eliminated. Pegan discourages cow's milk dairy products altogether.

MEDITERRANEAN DIET

The Mediterranean diet also focuses on heart health and has a few similar principles to the pegan diet. Both encourage higher amounts of vegetables, using olive oil and eating seafood regularly. From there, however, they differ. Mediterranean promotes vegetable oils, reduced sodium, higher intake of whole grains and strictly limiting red meat to just a few times per month. The pegan diet focuses on oils other than those that are vegetable-based and limited whole grains. While neither stresses that meat should be the most-consumed food, pegan prefers quality meat in moderation, whereas the Mediterranean diet specifically decreases red meat intake.

BOTTOM LINE

Overall, the pegan diet is based on well-founded principles that promote food quality with a generous intake of vegetables and omega-3 fatty acids. Within the confines of pegan, there is plenty of room for customizing parameters to account for individual health needs.

Ever since Dr. Hyman coined the term in 2014 it has grown into a popular eating plan that strikes a happy medium between the paleo diet and the vegan diet. In the next chapter, we will elaborate on the health benefits of eating a pegan diet and how it can improve specific health markers.

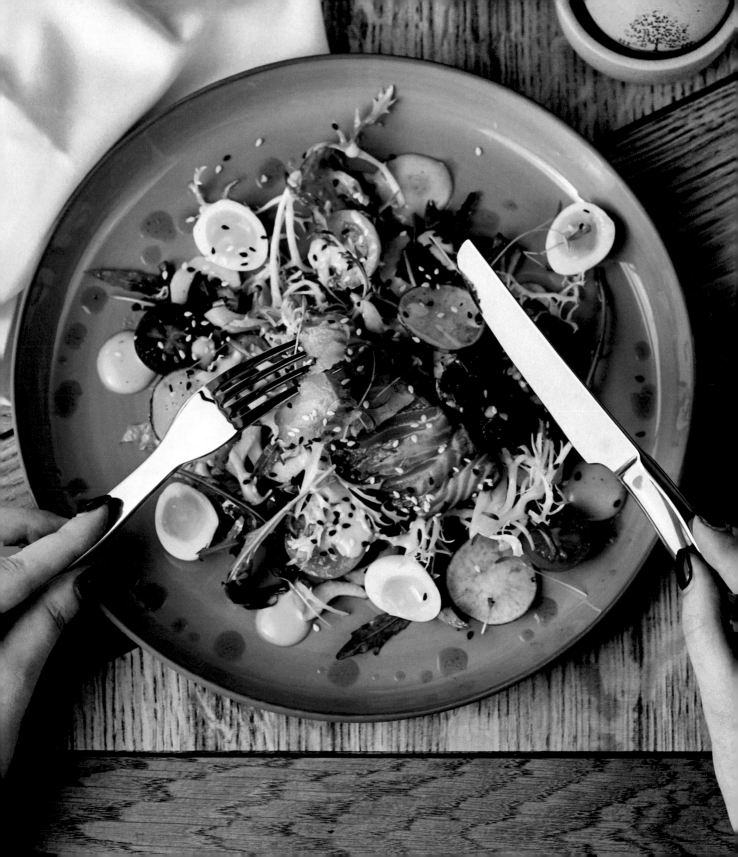

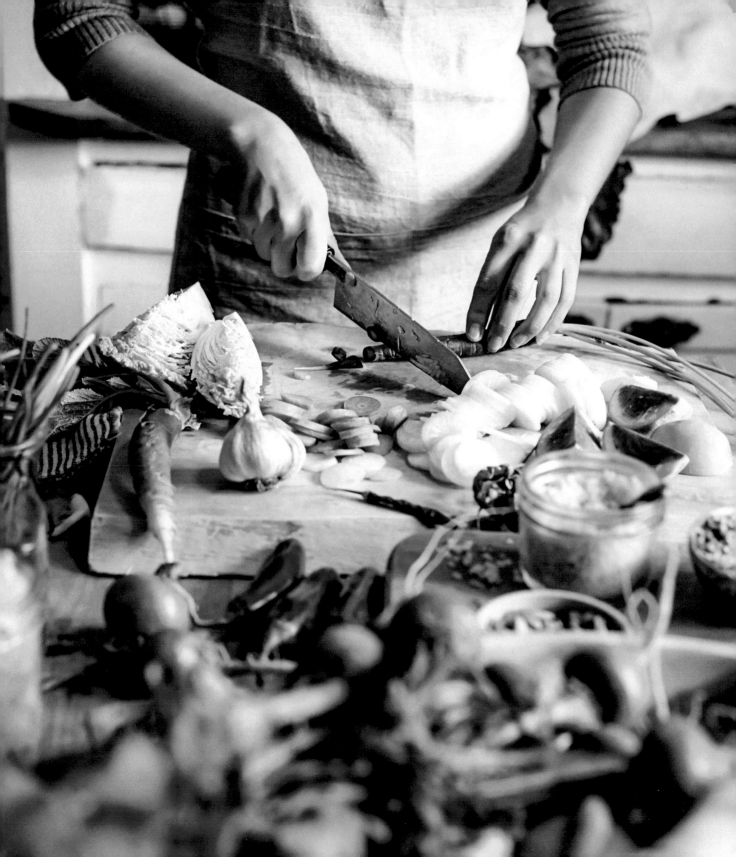

Why Pegan Is One of the Best Diets

Many diets are too strict to be sustainable over long periods of time, but the pegan diet's flexibility makes it easy to stick with for life.

MANY DIETARY protocols are restrictive, hard to follow and ultimately nutritionally incomplete. The pegan diet was created as a meeting point of positive research on two highly popular diets: paleo and vegan. Instead of pitting them against each other, pegan combines the best of both worlds and allows for a vegetable-heavy diet that still includes high-quality animal products.

Nutrition is essential for human health, but for many people, eating becomes an afterthought, a form of entertainment or a coping mechanism. American fast food and convenience products are devoid of whole ingredients and naturally occurring vitamins and minerals. The society we live in is obsessed with quick fixes and celebrity fads.

In 2019, Dr. Hyman explained how this diet isn't a trend or a short-lived fad. In a blog post on *MindBodyGreen*, Hyman wrote that pegan is not a "quick fix" meant to be followed for 10 or 30 days, only to return to your previous way of eating. Instead, he says: "After you reset your body, I recommend eating this way every single day. It is inclusive, not exclusive, and based on sound nutritional science and working with patients for more than 30 years."

People need to feel empowered in what they're eating—not stressed out or too busy to be present in the process. Understanding what the research shows and applying that to personal health is the foundation of a pegan plan.

LIMITATIONS OF NUTRITION RESEARCH

In his book *Food: What the Heck Should I Eat?*, Hyman writes about ending the confusion, insecurity and fear surrounding food choices. Real food, he says, is the best form of healing medicine on the planet, and should not be something that inspires arguments and confusion.

"Food is the most powerful drug on the planet. It can improve the expression of thousands of genes, balance dozens of hormones, optimize tens of thousands of protein networks, reduce inflammation and optimize your microbiome (gut flora) with every single bite," he says. Unfortunately, research about food and nutrition is still conflicting at times and open to interpretation—or worse, manipulation by food companies and manufacturers.

"Part of the reason we're so confused about what we should eat," Hyman says, "is that nutrition research is hard to conduct.... The results of nutritional studies are never as definitive as we might like them to be."

Nutritional studies are primarily conducted based on questionnaires and surveys of large groups—they typically ask people to recall from memory what they ate over a few-day time period or tally a general recollection of habits from the previous year. Most people are too busy or not fastidious enough to accurately represent their true dietary habits in these types of surveys. People tend to overreport or underreport their intake, resulting in skewed data.

It's also important to look at who funded the studies. Within the food industry, it's common to see agricultural giants or other food producers funding the studies that ultimately declare their product is healthy or that a competitive product is not. It's difficult for the average person to dig up original research from scientific and medical journals, let alone figure out who funded the studies or what biases the authors had.

With so much debate about what you should or shouldn't eat, an incredibly restrictive diet could cause more problems than it solves, which reinforces why a more balanced diet like pegan is such a solid choice. While the pegan diet encourages avoidance of cow's milk dairy products, as well as refined and processed foods, it allows for a wider inclusion of other food groups: meat, poultry, seafood, fruits and vegetables, grains, legumes, nuts and seeds.

Hyman—and most other nutrition professionals—argue that dietary choices need to be first and foremost customized to the person's individual needs. But within the realm of such broad food choices, a pegan program can help narrow the categories, while still providing a great deal of flexibility and customization.

RESEARCH ON PEGAN DIET BENEFITS

The principles of the pegan diet are backed by solid research showing that it can reduce chronic disease, improve overall health and lead to a longer life by combining the benefits of both the vegan and paleo diets.

ANTIOXIDANTS

One of the primary reasons the pegan diet promotes health is it focuses heavily on vegetable and fruit intake, suggesting 75 percent of the plate should be from fresh produce. Vegetables and fruits are rich in fiber, vitamins and minerals and contain plenty of antioxidants.

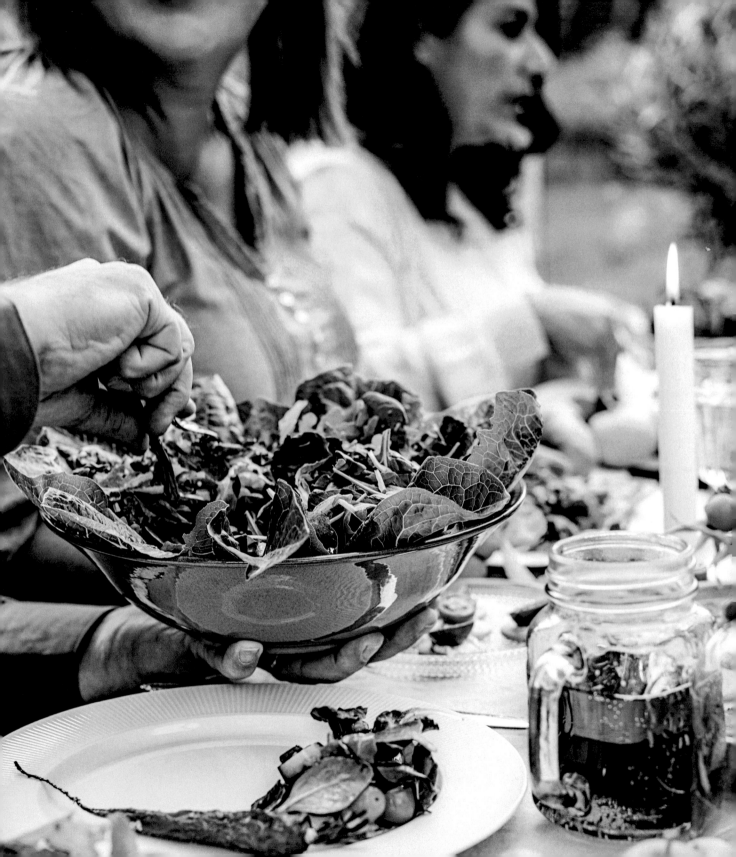

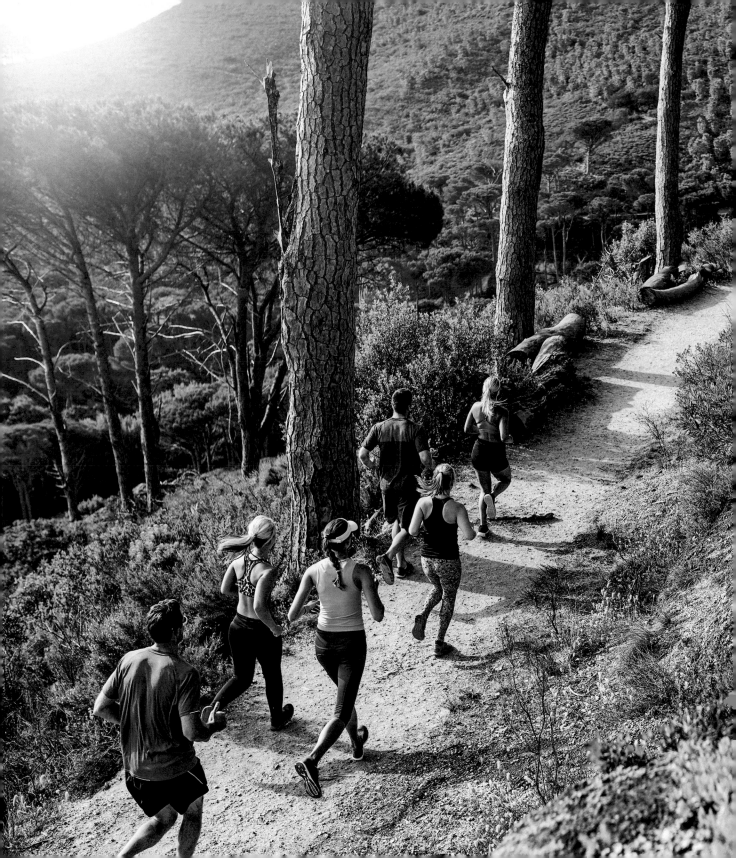

Antioxidants in the body fight oxidative stress which can cause cellular damage. When that occurs, it results in faster aging, cellular breakdown and DNA replication errors. By increasing the volume of antioxidants in the diet, it's possible to prevent or reverse this and boost cellular health.

BRAIN HEALTH

The modern fast food way of eating is destructive for brain health. Alzheimer's, dementia and other memory problems occur more frequently in people who have diabetes, excessive dietary sugar intake and an overall low-fat food approach.

Diets rich in fruits and vegetables help prevent memory loss, especially when they are eaten in the 20 years preceding the typical onset (so, in the 30s and 40s).

Generous intake of fruits and vegetables not only protects brain health physically, but it boosts mental health, improving overall feelings of wellness and happiness. Research from the University of Leeds found that even just one extra portion daily of fruits and vegetables had the same mental effect as 80 minutes of exercise in a month. While exercise is still important, of course, the mental boost of feeling better could improve motivation, resulting in more dedication to a fitness program and sticking with a healthy eating plan.

HEART HEALTH

While other diets focus specifically on supporting heart health or preventing heart disease, the pegan diet promotes this effortlessly thanks to the presence of so many antioxidants, omega-3 fats, fiber and a dramatically decreased intake of refined sugars and grains.

The higher intake of nutrients like potassium—which comes from foods like sweet potatoes, avocado, spinach, beans and bananas—could make pegan a diet that naturally supports reduced blood pressure. While most of the heart-healthy advice in the U.S. focuses on cutting sodium, boosting potassium intake is actually equally or more important. In fact, higher potassium intake from foods is associated with lower blood pressure regardless of what sodium intake is.

The typical Western diet is loaded with sodium and very low in potassium, but a pegan diet naturally avoids processed foods and promotes regular intake of foods that are naturally rich in potassium.

LUNG HEALTH

Fruits and vegetables are an abundant source of vitamin C, which is an antioxidant nutrient that supports healthy lungs. Apples and tomatoes especially have been shown to be preventive and protective against respiratory infections.

Polyunsaturated fatty acids, like omega-3 fats EPA and DHA, are also associated with a lowered risk of bronchial hyperresponsiveness in asthma and other lung sensitivity. Excess intake of omega-6 fats, without enough omega-3s to counterbalance, results in an increased risk for asthmatic complications.

INFLAMMATION

The high volume of fresh produce on a pegan diet leads to a direct reduction in inflammatory processes. Inflammation is often a trigger for chronic disease, swelling, pain and even cancer.

Omega-3 fats are so potent at reducing inflammation that they can cut certain markers, like C-reactive protein, in cancer patients. C-reactive protein, or CRP, is commonly used to assess cardiovascular risk and systemic inflammation. Because a vegan diet alone excludes animal-based omega-3 fats, like salmon and mackerel, paleo diets are often superior at reducing inflammatory markers. However, when paired with the significant body of research illustrating how fresh produce downgrades inflammation by fighting oxidative stress in the body, it's clear both elements are needed to truly protect overall health.

WEIGHT LOSS

Diets that encourage a higher intake of plant-based foods versus animal foods are highly protective against obesity and promote natural weight loss. Research from the University of Navarra found that those who ate plenty of plant-based foods like vegetables, fruits and even some whole grains reduced the risk of obesity by nearly half. This type of plant-based diet also helps protect against diabetes and heart disease.

However, research also supports low-carb, high-fat diets for weight loss and the reduction of body fat. A pegan diet is the best of both worlds, pairing high vegetable and fruit intake with restricted intake of starchy carbs like grains and promoting a moderate intake of protein and healthy, anti-inflammatory fats.

For the pegan diet to promote weight loss, it does not have to be calorie-restricted or portion-controlled, with the exception of always using meat, grains, nuts and seeds as sides and giving most of your plate space to vegetables and fruits.

AND MORE

This is far from an exhaustive list of all the benefits pegan eating has to offer. Diets rich in whole, unprocessed foods also promote more satiety, a healthier relationship with food, reduced cancer risk and improved digestion.

HOW TO EFFECTIVELY AND SAFELY LOSE WEIGHT FOLLOWING A PEGAN PROGRAM

Whenever you're starting a new dietary program, it's always smart to check in with your doctor. Prior to beginning a dietary shift, having baseline bloodwork done—especially when it comes to inflammatory markers, lipids, glucose, insulin and more—can allow you to gauge your progress with how the diet is helping you achieve your goals and improving your overall health. Pounds lost on the scale are not the only markers of wellness, and sometimes improvements in other health markers happen before the weight starts to come off.

As Hyman has said, the pegan diet is about individualizing the approach, not following a cookie-cutter system. Aspects of the pegan diet may not be right for you if you are diabetic or have other health conditions. This is where checking in with your personal medical team can be helpful and can set you up for success.

Over time, your dietary needs might change as well. Pegan can be flexible, with a wide

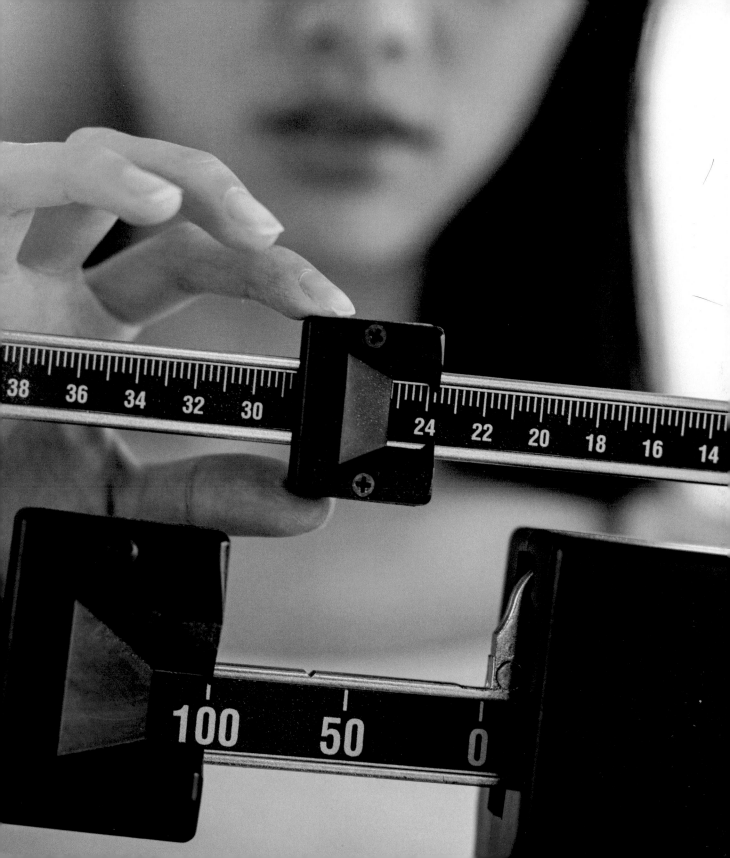

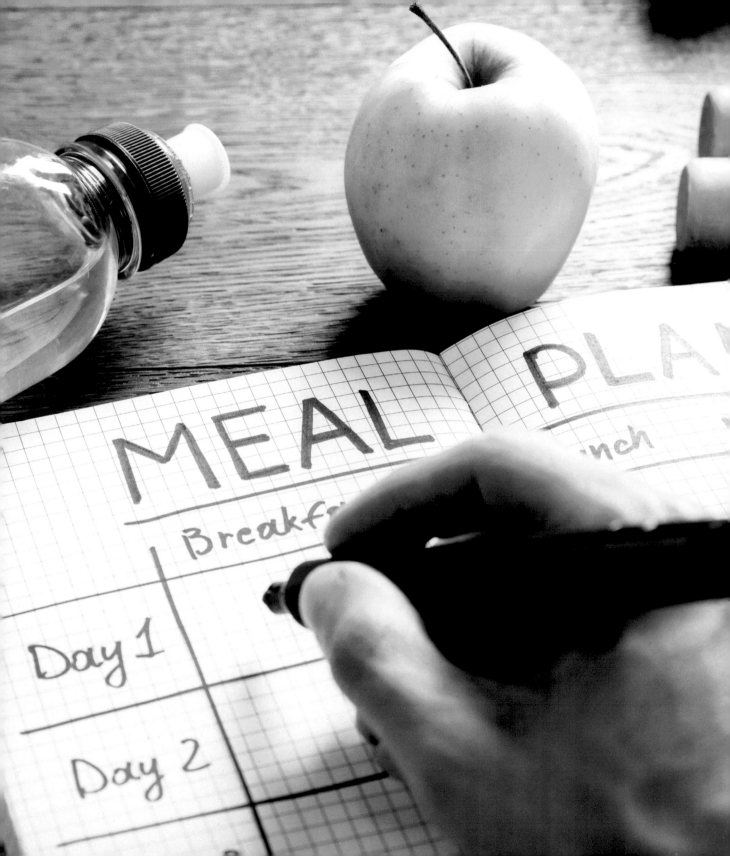

range of customization allowable within the guidelines.

Most importantly, pegan eating is not about deprivation or exclusion, but rather nourishment and inclusion. Avoiding processed and sugary foods is important—but this doesn't mean you have to feel deprived. There are many ways to create delicious meals, snacks and even treats from pegan-friendly foods, as you'll see in this book's recipes.

HOW TO GET STARTED ON A PEGAN DIET

Getting started on a pegan diet can happen in a few different ways. This book provides more than 125 recipes to get you started, as well as a meal plan that covers four weeks of eating. If you want to dive right in, start with the meal plan.

But you can also pick and choose recipes from this book to get used to the pegan diet for a few weeks or a month to dip your toe into the water of this new way of eating. You'll find the recipes are not only easy to follow, but they're delicious and don't taste like "boring diet food" at all.

Pegan can be something you follow exclusively or you can try an 80/20 approach, meaning you would eat pegan during the week, for example, and eat whatever you want on weekends. The benefits of pegan eating don't only happen when you exclusively follow the plan, although the more meals you devote to this mentality, the healthier you will arguably be.

If jumping into a month-long meal plan seems too overwhelming, try having one pegan day a week and gradually work your way up to all seven days. As you learn the dietary principles and they become second nature, you won't need to think so hard and you'll be able to effortlessly work it into your daily routine.

Having a support network for a new way of eating can also improve success rates and overall enjoyment. If your partner or family members aren't eating the pegan diet with you, find a friend to join along. You can swap meals and trade tips on food prep and recipe favorites, and you'll motivate each other to keep at it.

The pegan diet, because it is not calorie-restricted, is safe and healthy for people of all ages, including pregnant and breastfeeding women. While personal advice from your doctor trumps everything, pegan is safe because it does not go to any extremes and encourages plenty of real, whole foods with minimal processing.

BOTTOM LINE

The pegan diet is a nutrient-dense food plan that pairs the health benefits of paleo with those of the vegan diet. By matching these two seemingly polar opposites, you're actually receiving a more well-rounded food plan than those who follow one extreme or the other.

Hyman has been recommending the pegan way of eating to his patients for years, and he personally eats it himself. Many nutritionists have found this same middle ground between what feels like fad dietary approaches, citing the excellent health benefits of both methods.

The benefit of a pegan diet is it can be fully customized to each individual's needs, resulting in dozens, if not hundreds, of different potential ways to harness its power. Read on to determine which one is right for you.

Pegan Cheat Sheet

An at-a-glance guide to what you should be eating.

EAT A LOT
Non-starchy vegetables
Low-glycemic fruits (berries, kiwis, oranges, etc.)
Eggs
Fresh, low-mercury seafood (salmon, mackerel, sardines, anchovies, etc.)

EAT A MODERATE AMOUNT
Low-glycemic grains, such as black rice or quinoa (up to ½ cup per meal)
Beans and legumes (up to 1 cup per day)
Organic, grass-fed meat and poultry (up to 4 to 6 ounces per meal)
Healthy fats (olive oil, avocado oil, coconut oil, ghee, butter)

EAT A LITTLE
Starchy vegetables
High-glycemic fruits (grapes, melons, cherries, etc.)
Nuts and seeds
Goat or sheep's milk dairy

OCCASIONAL TREATS
Dried fruits
Juices
Sugar
Alcohol (up to 2 to 3 servings per week)

AVOID
Processed foods
Cow's milk dairy (except occasional butter or ghee)
Vegetable oils (canola, corn, soybean, sunflower, etc.)

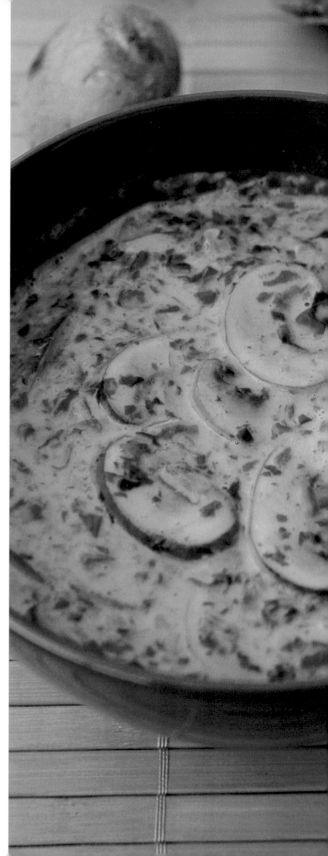

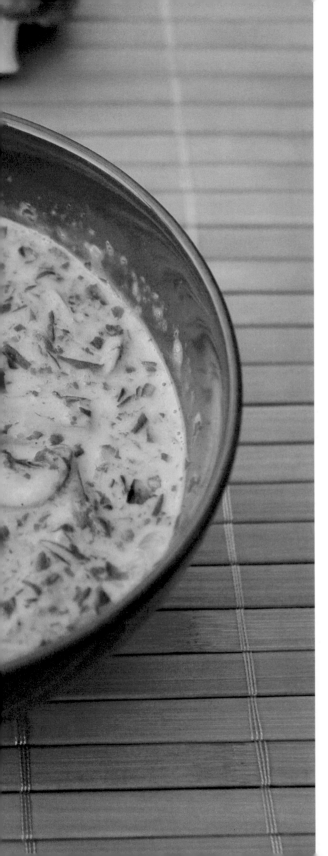

The Pegan Pantry

Make food prep easier by stocking your pantry with these popular pegan-friendly foods.

VEGETABLES
Beets
Broccoli
Brussels
  sprouts
Leeks
Onions
Garlic
Ginger
Bok choy
Squash
Cauliflower
Tomatoes
Spinach
Green beans
Kale
Chard
Peppers
Cucumbers
Turnips
Sweet potatoes
Carrots
Radishes
Asparagus

FRUITS
Bananas
Oranges
Grapefruit
Kiwi fruit
Pears
Nectarines

Blueberries
Raspberries
Strawberries
Avocados
Lemons
Limes

PROTEIN
Eggs
Organic,
  grass-fed
  meat
Low-mercury
  seafood
Tofu
Tempeh
Edamame

HEALTHY FATS
Olive oil
Avocado oil
Coconut oil
Ghee
Nuts
Seeds

STARCHES
Black rice
Red rice
Quinoa
Soba noodles

Beans
Lentils

DAIRY
Organic, grass-
  fed butter
Ghee
Yogurt
Kefir
Goat's cheese

MISCELLANEOUS
Vinegars
Fresh herbs
Broth
Tahini
Almond milk
Coconut milk

SUPPLEMENTS
Vitamin D
Vitamin B12

SWEETS
Honey
Maple syrup
Dark chocolate

- APRICOTS
- PLUMS
- RASPBERRIES
- NECTARINES
- PEACHES
- PLUMS
- FIGS
- BLUEBERRIES

28-Day Pegan Meal Plan

Dive right into the pegan diet with four weeks of delicious breakfast, lunch and dinner recipes.

pegan meal plan
week one

DAY	BREAKFAST	LUNCH	DINNER
1	Avocado Breakfast Bake (p.37)	Salmon Salad Appetizers (p.70) with Arugula Cucumber Gazpacho (p.101)	Braised Short Ribs (p.153) with Pan-Roasted Radishes (p.125)
2	Start-Your-Day Smoothie Bowl (p.63)	Roasted Eggplants (p.70) with Guacamole Deviled Eggs (p.76)	Asian Skillet Salmon (p.160) with Cauliflower Rice (p.129) and Roasted Bok Choy (p.130)
3	Blueberry Nut Millet Porridge (p.40)	Buffalo Chicken Soup (p.97)	Roasted Garlic and Herb Millet Polenta (p.157) with Mexican Street Asparagus (p.141)
4	Breakfast Bake (p.43)	Grilled Radicchio and Pear Salad with Warm Bacon Dressing (p.112) with Beef-Wrapped Vegetable Bundles (p.83)	Blackberry Lamb Chop (p.154) with Beet Noodles with Red Pepper Pesto (p.137)
5	Morning Mash (p.47)	Butternut Squash Soup with Cajun Prawns (p.107)	Slow Cooker Pulled Pork (p.172) with Apple Cucumber Coleslaw (p.132)
6	Coconut Matcha Kiwi Parfait (p.47)	Arugula, Raspberry and Hazelnut Salad (p.115) with Grilled Zucchini and Tomato Roll-Ups (p.74)	Vegetable and Mussels Bowl (p.160) with Five-Spice Butternut Squash Ribbons (p.134)
7	Breakfast Bowl (p.44)	Lemon Ginger Avgolemono (p.110)	Hot Chicken Wings Piccata (p.158) with Roasted Tomato Zucchini Boats (p.138)

DAY	BREAKFAST	LUNCH	DINNER
8	Very Berry Protein Pancakes (p.48)	Easy Vegetable Bean Soup (p.97)	Fettuccine Alfredo (p.155) with Pan-Fried Spicy Oyster Mushrooms (p.142)
9	Blueberry Nut Overnight Chia Pudding (p.40)	Summer Salad (p.98)	Salmon Salad Sliders (p.159) with Vegetable Fries with Lemon Garlic Gremolata (p.126)
10	Breakfast Salmon Scramble (p.54)	Mini Sliders with Brussels Sprout Buns (p.69) with Tri-Beet Salad (p.117)	Mediterranean Vegetable Shrimp Scampi (p.170) with Cauliflower Rice (p.129)
11	Crab Crepes (p.51) with fresh fruit	Spaghetti Squash Cakes (p.84) with Vegetable and Shrimp Ceviche (p.87)	Buffalo Cauliflower Lettuce Cups (p.162) with Roasted Beets with Goat Cheese (p.133)
12	Sausage Breakfast Frittata (p.52)	Brussels Sprout and Beet Salad with Lemon Poppy Seed Dressing (p.99) with Grilled Green Oysters (p.78)	Sweet Potato Black Bean Chili (p.187)
13	Granola Bars (p.56) with fresh fruit	Sweet Potato Toast (p.82)	Beef and Broccoli (p.183) with Cauliflower Fried Black Rice (p.136)
14	Breakfast Bento Box (p.46)	Vegetable-Stuffed Artichokes (p.91)	Shrimp Dinner Pockets (p.178) with Red Rice Risotto (p.129)

week three

DAY	BREAKFAST	LUNCH	DINNER
15	Eggs and Garden Vegetable Spread (p.55)	Kale, Blood Orange and Pomegranate Salad with Ginger Carrot Dressing (p.105) with Steamed Chicken and Vegetable Pinwheels (p.90)	Swedish Meatballs (p.184) with Cauliflower Rice (p.129)
16	Orange Pomegranate Crepes (p.60)	Vegetable Quinoa Salad (p.121) with Beef-Wrapped Vegetable Bundles (p.83)	Chicken and Pineapple Skewers (p.171) with Sesame Ginger–Glazed Soba Noodles (p.134)
17	Morning Mash (p.47)	Asian Skillet Salmon (p.160) with Romaine Wedge Salad with Lemon, Basil and Flaxseed Dressing (p.108)	Artisan Tomato Sandwich with Healthy Sandwich Spread (p.182) with Carrot Ginger Soup (p.115)
18	Omelet-Stuffed Peppers (p.59)	Hearty Mushroom and Spinach Soup (p.118) with Grilled Zucchini and Tomato Roll-Ups (p.74)	Skillet Braised Salmon and Vegetables (p.169)
19	Breakfast Salmon Scramble (p.54)	Butternut Squash Soup with Cajun Prawns (p.107)	Slow Cooker Pulled Pork (p.172) with Roasted and Mashed Turnips (p.145) and Sweet-and-Sour Swiss Chard (p.148)
20	Very Berry Protein Pancakes (p.48)	Black Rice Cakes with Scallops and Leek Cream Sauce (p.68) with Mini Sliders with Brussels Sprout Buns (p.69)	Stuffed Poblano Peppers (p.163) with Roasted Squash with Tahini Sauce (p.147)
21	Avocado Breakfast Bake (p.37)	Buffalo Chicken Soup (p.97)	Stuffed Meatloaf (p.172) with Vegetable Chop (p.146)

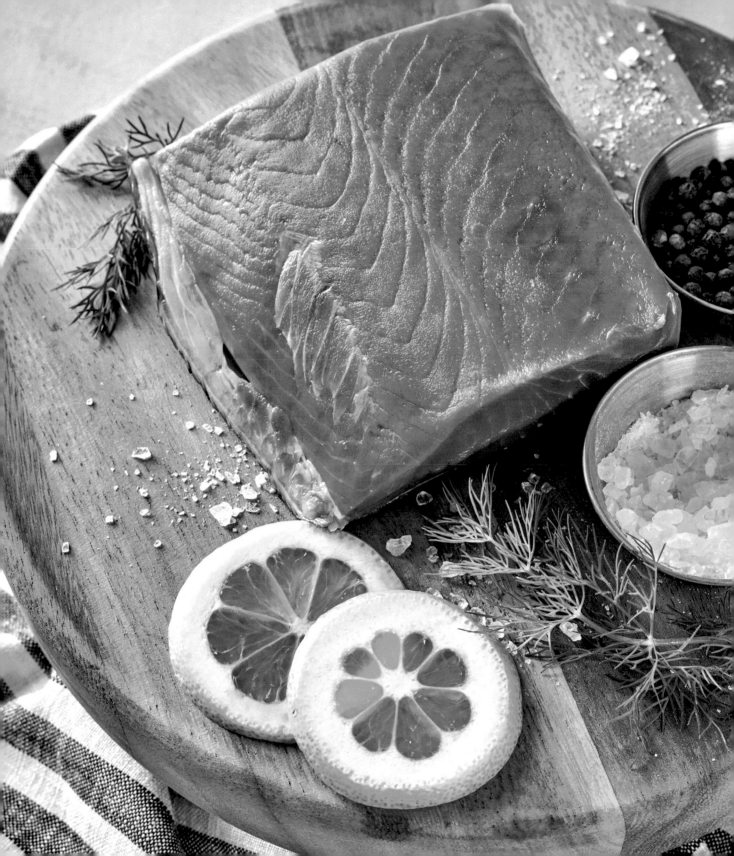

week four

DAY	BREAKFAST	LUNCH	DINNER
22	Sausage Breakfast Frittata (p.52)	Brussels Sprout Salad (p.102) with Spicy Coconut Shrimp with Pegan Cocktail Sauce (p.73)	Slow Cooker Chicken Cacciatore (p.175) with Tri-Beet Salad (p.117)
23	Blueberry Nut Millet Porridge (p.40)	Steamed Chicken and Vegetable Pinwheels (p.90)	Salmon Salad Sliders (p.159) with Apple Cucumber Coleslaw (p.132)
24	Breakfast Bowl (p.44)	Sweet Potato Toast (p.82)	Mushroom Stew (p.167) with Red Rice Risotto (p.129)
25	Granola Bars (p.56) with sliced avocado	Frisée, Grapefruit and Long Bean Salad with Warm Anchovy, Orange and Herb Dressing (p.104) with Fried Anchovies (p.93)	Quinoa and Sweet Potato Burger (p.165) with Cucumber Spiral Salad (p.109)
26	Start-Your-Day Smoothie Bowl (p.63)	Summer Salad (p.98)	Stuffed Eggplant (p.176) with Vegetable Fries with Lemon Garlic Gremolata (p.126)
27	Blueberry Nut Overnight Chia Pudding (p.40)	Easy Vegetable Bean Soup (p.97)	Orange Pepper Pesto–Stuffed Roasted Cabbage Steaks (p.166) with Beet Noodles with Red Pepper Pesto (p.137)
28	Bacon and Egg Cauliflower Breakfast Pizza (p.39)	Lemon Ginger Avgolemono (p.110)	Chicken and Pineapple Skewers (p.171)

substitutions

If you're short on an ingredient or want to make a favorite recipe more pegan-friendly, try one of these swaps listed below.

1 EGG

FOR BAKING

1 tablespoon flaxseed or chia seed + 3 tablespoons water, mixed and refrigerated for 30 minutes

———

¼ cup unsweetened organic applesauce, pumpkin purée mashed organic bananas

———

¼ cup puréed silken organic tofu

FOR SCRAMBLED EGGS

¼ cup firm or extra-firm tofu, crumbled

BUTTER

FOR SAUTÉING AND SAUCES

1:1 olive oil, coconut oil, ghee, cocoa butter or coconut butter

FOR BAKING

1:1 almond butter, applesauce, mashed bananas or avocados, or pumpkin purée

COW'S MILK CHEESE

Goat or sheep cheese, such as fresh goat's cheese, pecorino, Manchego, halloumi or feta

YOGURT

1:1 sheep or goat yogurt

SOUR CREAM

1:1 sheep or goat yogurt

MILK

1:1 almond or soy milk

FLOUR

1:1 almond flour

CORNSTARCH

1:1 arrowroot or tapioca

BACON

1:1 turkey bacon

VANILLA BEAN CAVIAR

1:1 unsweetened vanilla bean extract

conversions

VOLUME

¼ teaspoon	=	1 mL
½ teaspoon	=	2 mL
1 teaspoon	=	5 mL
1 tablespoon	=	15 mL
¼ cup	=	50 mL
⅓ cup	=	75 mL
½ cup	=	125 mL
⅔ cup	=	150 mL
¾ cup	=	175 mL
1 cup	=	250 mL
1 quart	=	1 liter
1½ quarts	=	1.5 liters
2 quarts	=	2 liters
2½ quarts	=	2.5 liters
3 quarts	=	3 liters
4 quarts	=	4 liters

WEIGHT

1 ounce	=	30 grams
2 ounces	=	55 grams
3 ounces	=	85 grams
4 ounces (¼ pound)	=	115 grams
8 ounces (½ pound)	=	225 grams
16 ounces (1 pound)	=	445 grams
2 pounds	=	910 grams

LENGTH

⅛ inch	=	3 mm
¼ inch	=	6 mm
½ inch	=	13 mm
¾ inch	=	19 mm
1 inch	=	2.5 cm
2 inches	=	5 cm

TEMPERATURES

FAHRENHEIT		CELSIUS
32°	=	0°
212°	=	100°
250°	=	120°
275°	=	140°
300°	=	150°
325°	=	160°
350°	=	180°
375°	=	190°
400°	=	200°
425°	=	220°
450°	=	230°
475°	=	240°
500°	=	260°

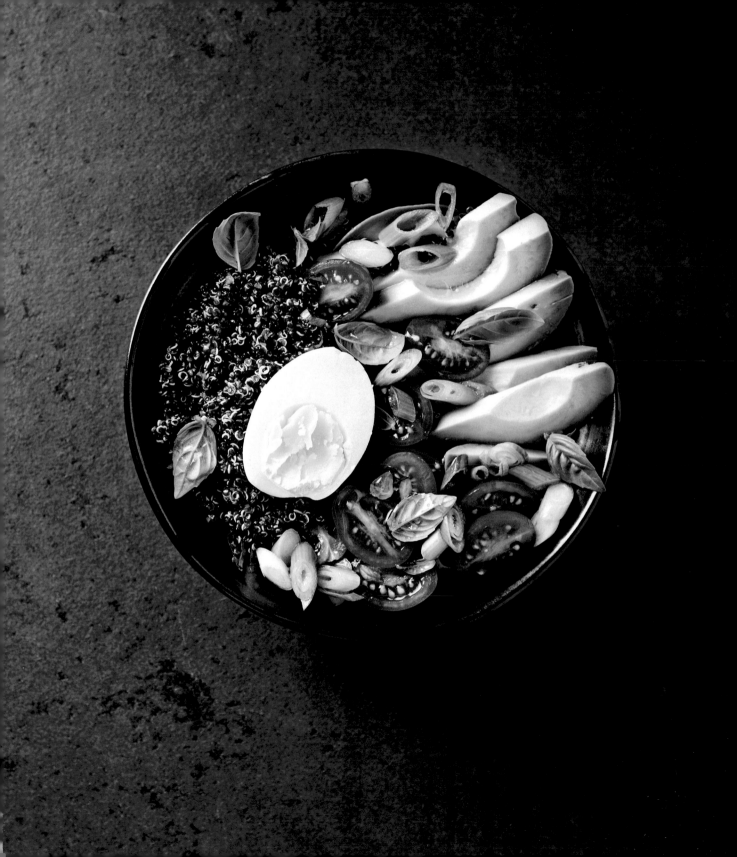

breakfast

START YOUR DAY WITH FILLING, NUTRITIOUS FOODS.

Avocado Breakfast Bake 37

Bacon and Egg Cauliflower Breakfast Pizza 39

Candied Bacon 39

Blueberry Nut Millet Porridge 40

Blueberry Nut Overnight Chia Pudding 40

Breakfast Bake 43

Breakfast Bowl 44

Breakfast Bento Box 46

Morning Mash 47

Coconut Matcha Kiwi Parfait 47

Very Berry Protein Pancakes 48

Crab Crepes 51

Sausage Breakfast Frittata 52

Breakfast Salmon Scramble 54

Eggs and Garden Vegetable Spread 55

Granola Bars 56

Omelet-Stuffed Peppers 59

Orange Pomegranate Crepes 60

Sweet Potato and Pulled Pork Eggs Benedict 62

Start-Your-Day Smoothie Bowl 63

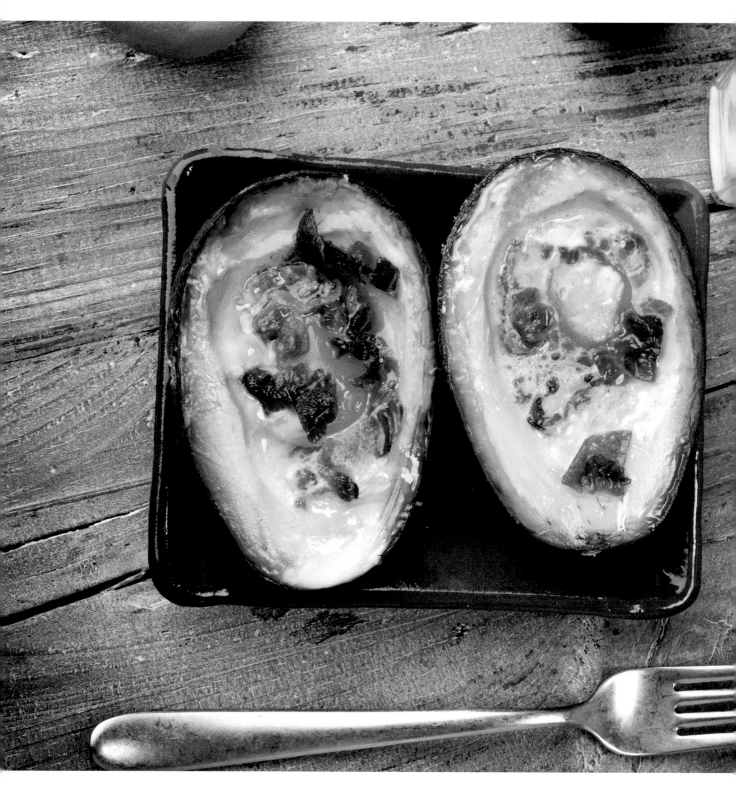

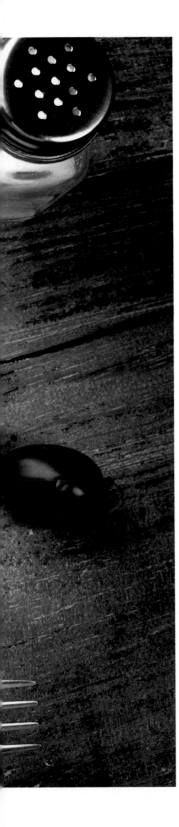

AVOCADO BREAKFAST BAKE

Sometimes the simplest things are the best. Avocados and eggs are a classic combination, and the prosciutto adds a salty and crunchy kick to this easy dish.

INGREDIENTS

- 2 **large ripe avocados**
- 4 **slices prosciutto**
- 4 **eggs**
- **Salt and pepper, to taste**

DIRECTIONS

SERVES 4

Preheat oven to 375 degrees F.

Cut the avocados in half and remove seeds. Place the avocados in a baking dish. Top each avocado with a slice of prosciutto and push the prosciutto into the pit well, letting the edges raise up so they get crispy. If the well is not large enough for the egg, scoop some avocado out. Crack an egg in each well and season with salt and pepper.

Place in preheated oven and cook for 15 minutes, or until the eggs are cooked and the yolk is still runny.

PER SERVING: Calories: 253, Fat: 20g, Protein: 12g, Sodium: 327mg, Fiber: 5.9g, Carbohydrates: 8.4g, Sugar: 1.1g

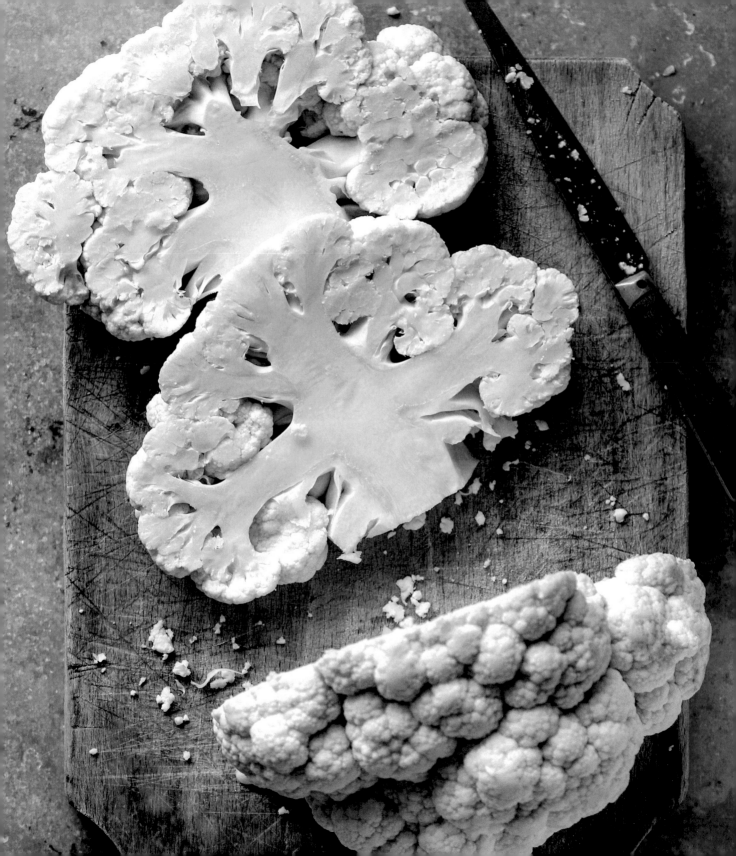

BACON AND EGG CAULIFLOWER BREAKFAST PIZZA

The "make everything out of cauliflower" craze is popular for a reason—cauliflower really is a perfect vessel in so many ways, from rice to crusts to steaks! This recipe skips the classic cauliflower pizza crust and instead uses steaks to make a filling and rustic breakfast pizza.

INGREDIENTS

DIRECTIONS

SERVES 4

- 1 large cauliflower, sliced into 4 steaks
- 2 tablespoons olive oil
- ½ teaspoon sea salt
- ½ teaspoon freshly ground black pepper
- 8 slices bacon
- 2 cups Garden Vegetable Spread (page 55)
- 3 ounces goat cheese, crumbled
- 4 eggs

Preheat oven to 350 degrees F.

Brush the cauliflower steaks with oil and season with salt and pepper. Place the remaining oil onto a sheet pan and place the steaks onto the sheet pan. Place in the oven and cook for about 20 minutes, or until just fork-tender.

Meanwhile, in a frying pan, cook the bacon on medium heat until browned and crispy. Drain on paper towels.

Take cauliflower steaks out of the oven and top each with Garden Vegetable Spread, cheese and bacon and crack an egg on each. Place it back in the oven and bake until the egg is cooked and the yolk is still runny.

PER SERVING: Calories: 424, Fat: 31g, Protein: 21g, Sodium: 692mg, Fiber: 8.5g, Carbohydrates: 17g, Sugar: 6.4g

CANDIED BACON

This sweet and salty combination can be served at breakfast or dessert—try a piece broken up over ice cream or pudding.

INGREDIENTS

DIRECTIONS

SERVES 4

- ½ pound bacon
- ½ cup maple syrup
- ½ cup pistachios, crushed

Preheat oven to 375 degrees F.

Place bacon on a wire rack over a sheet pan. Brush the bacon evenly with syrup and coat with nuts. Place in the oven and cook for 10 to 15 minutes, or until bacon is browned and crisp.

PER SERVING: Calories: 485, Fat: 30g, Protein: 20g, Sodium: 912mg, Fiber: 0.8g, Carbohydrates: 29g, Sugar: 28g

BLUEBERRY NUT MILLET PORRIDGE

You won't miss oatmeal after trying this millet porridge!
Make it your own by mixing in your favorite flavors.

INGREDIENTS

- 2 cups uncooked millet
- 2 teaspoons almond butter
- 4 cups unsweetened almond milk
- 2 cups water
- ¼ teaspoon sea salt
- 1 tablespoon cinnamon
- ¼ teaspoon vanilla bean caviar
- 2 tablespoons honey
- 2 cups blueberries
- ½ cup almonds
- 2 tablespoons hemp seeds

DIRECTIONS

In a coffee grinder or food processor, pulse millet until half the grains are broken.

Add butter to a medium saucepan over medium-low heat. Stir in the millet and lightly toast for 2 to 3 minutes.

Add milk, water, salt, cinnamon, vanilla and honey. Bring to a simmer, cover and cook for 15 to 20 minutes, or until grains are soft, stirring occasionally. Add more milk if needed.

Top the porridge with blueberries, toasted almonds and hemp seeds.

PER SERVING: Calories: 361, Fat: 17g, Protein: 11g, Sodium: 230mg, Fiber: 7.1g, Carbohydrates: 47g, Sugar: 17g

SERVES 4

BLUEBERRY NUT OVERNIGHT CHIA PUDDING

Like overnight oats, chia pudding is perfect for prepping the night before, and the potential flavor combinations are endless. Experiment and come up with your own favorites!

INGREDIENTS

- ½ cup chia seeds
- 1½ cups fresh blueberries
- 1½ cups slivered almonds
- 2 tablespoons cinnamon
- 4 teaspoons honey
- 3–4 cups unsweetened almond milk

DIRECTIONS

In four glasses or mason jars, layer each container with chia seeds, blueberries, nuts, cinnamon and honey until all the ingredients are used. Fill each with almond milk, leaving about 1 inch free on top. Place in the refrigerator overnight.

PER SERVING: Calories: 500, Fat: 36g, Protein: 16g, Sodium: 121mg, Fiber: 17g, Carbohydrates: 37g, Sugar: 14g

SERVES 4

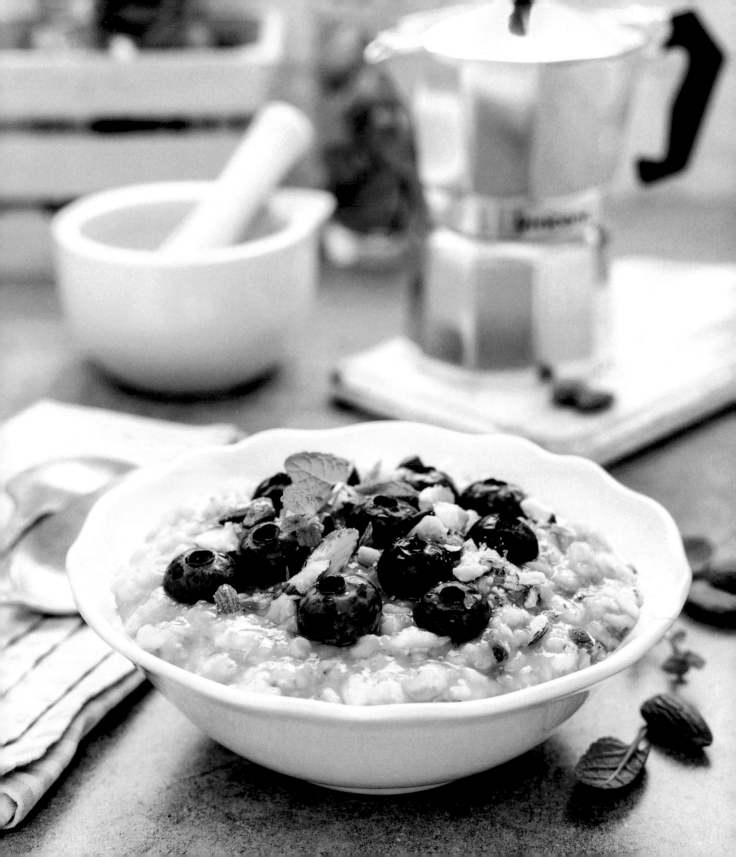

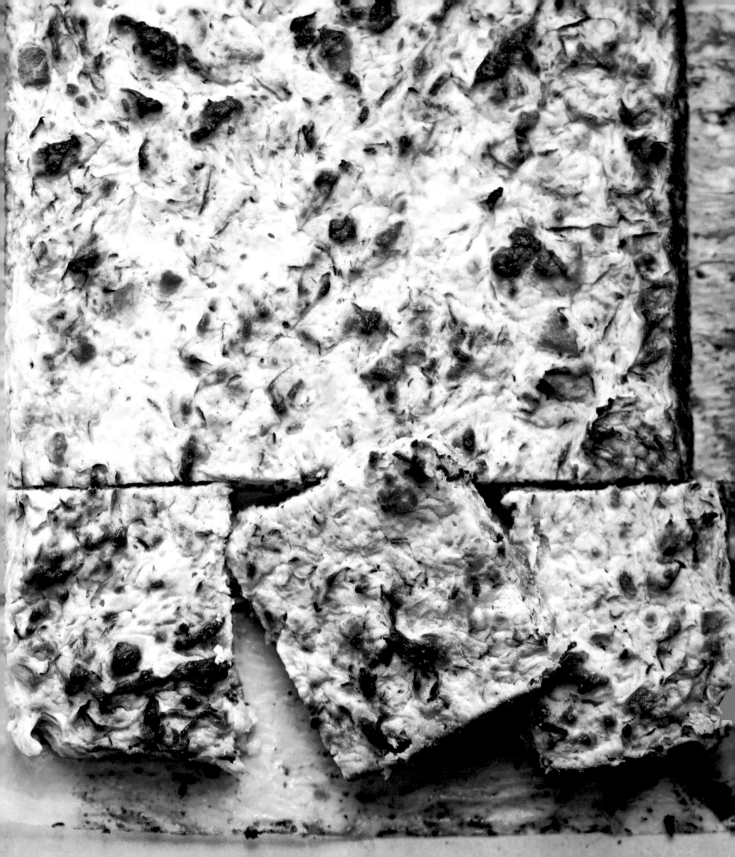

BREAKFAST BAKE

Breakfast bakes are perfect for when you're entertaining a crowd.
This recipe can easily be scaled up to feed as many people as you need!

INGREDIENTS

- ½ pound bacon
- 1 pound fingerling potatoes, diced
- 1 red pepper, diced
- 1 onion, diced
- 8 eggs
- ½ pint ripe grape tomatoes, quartered
- 2 tablespoons fresh chives, sliced
- ½ teaspoon sea salt
- ½ teaspoon freshly ground black pepper
- 2 cups salsa
- 2 avocados, sliced

DIRECTIONS

SERVES 4

Preheat oven to 350 degrees F.

In a medium pan on medium heat, cook the bacon until browned and crisp. Drain on paper towels.

Take 1 tablespoon of bacon grease from the pan and set aside. Place the potatoes into the same pan and cook until crisp and almost fork-tender. In the same pan, add the reserved bacon grease and cook the red pepper and onion until soft, about 4 to 5 minutes. Set aside.

Cut the bacon into bite-size pieces.

In a medium bowl, mix together the eggs, tomatoes, chives and bacon. Season with salt and pepper.

Place the potato mixture in an oven-safe baking dish. Top with the egg mixture and place in a preheated oven.

Cook for 20 minutes, or until eggs are cooked through. Cut the egg bake into pieces and serve topped with salsa and sliced avocado.

PER SERVING: Calories: 824, Fat: 52g, Protein: 38g, Sodium: 1,896mg, Fiber: 16g, Carbohydrates: 46g, Sugar: 14g

BREAKFAST BOWL

This start-your-day dish is packed with protein from the quinoa, eggs and prosciutto, guaranteeing you'll be satisfied until lunch.

INGREDIENTS	DIRECTIONS	SERVES 4

INGREDIENTS

- 1¼ cups uncooked quinoa
- 2½ cups water
- ¼ teaspoon sea salt
- 4 eggs
- 4 small clusters vine tomatoes
- 2 avocados
- 4 slices prosciutto

DIRECTIONS

Pour the quinoa into a fine mesh colander and rinse under water.

Combine the quinoa and salted water in a saucepan. Bring the mixture to a boil over medium-high heat, then lower the heat to a simmer. Cook until the quinoa has absorbed all of the water, about 15 to 20 minutes. Remove the pot from heat, cover and let the quinoa steam for 5 minutes. Remove the lid and fluff the quinoa with a fork.

Bring a second saucepan of water to a boil over medium-high heat. Use a slotted spoon to carefully lower the eggs into the boiling water. Lower heat to a simmer and cook the eggs for 6 minutes. Remove the eggs and place in a bath of cold water for 2 minutes, then peel the eggs.

Preheat a pan over medium heat. Add oil and cook the tomatoes until slightly charred and softened. Cut avocados in half lengthwise, remove the pits and cut slices into the avocado. Scoop out the avocado with a spoon.

Cut the eggs in half. Divide the quinoa into four serving bowls and arrange the tomatoes, eggs, avocados and prosciutto evenly on top of the quinoa.

PER SERVING: Calories: 501, Fat: 25g, Protein: 23g, Sodium: 441mg, Fiber: 14g, Carbohydrates: 52g, Sugar: 5.6g

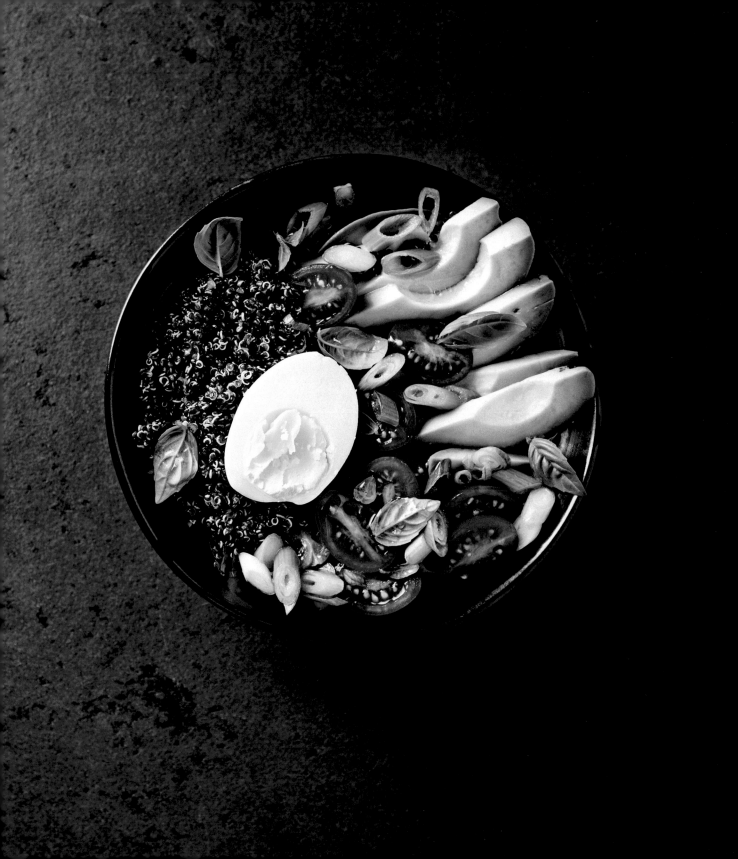

BREAKFAST BENTO BOX

Bento boxes are already a popular choice for lunch—why not use them to prepare your breakfasts, too?

INGREDIENTS **DIRECTIONS** SERVES 4

- 1 cup blueberries
- 1 cup raspberries
- 1 cup strawberries
- 4 eggs
- 4 Granola Bars (page 56)
- 2 cups sheep's yogurt

Wash and dry the berries.

Make perfect hard-boiled eggs: Place the eggs in a pot and cover with cold water by 1 inch. Bring to a boil, cover, remove from the heat and set aside for 8 to 10 minutes. Place the eggs in ice water to cool, then peel.

Evenly divide all the ingredients between four boxes.

Note: You can crumble your granola bar over your yogurt if desired.

PER SERVING: Calories: 957, Fat: 71g, Protein: 26g, Sodium: 124mg, Fiber: 13g, Carbohydrates: 75g, Sugar: 50g

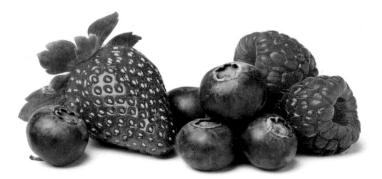

MORNING MASH

This "morning mash" comes together quickly on busy mornings, especially if you have pre-made hard-boiled eggs handy.

INGREDIENTS	DIRECTIONS	SERVES 1-2

INGREDIENTS

- 1 avocado, chopped
- 2 large hard-boiled eggs, diced
- 1 ripe tomato, chopped
- Himalayan pink salt

DIRECTIONS

Mix all ingredients together in a bowl and season with Himalayan pink salt.

PER SERVING: Calories: 272, Fat: 20g, Protein: 10g, Sodium: 78mg, Fiber: 9.6g, Carbohydrates: 16g, Sugar: 6.5g

COCONUT MATCHA KIWI PARFAIT

Switch up your regular yogurt with some exciting new tropical flavors! To make this breakfast feel extra-decadent, serve in martini glasses.

INGREDIENTS — **DIRECTIONS** — **SERVES 4**

INGREDIENTS

- 8 kiwis
- 1 cup sheep's yogurt
- 1 tablespoon honey
- Zest of 1 lime, plus juice of ½ lime
- 1 teaspoon matcha green tea powder
- ½ cup shaved coconut, toasted
- 4 sprigs mint

DIRECTIONS

Peel kiwis. With a small melon-baller, make kiwi balls from the kiwis.

In a small bowl, mix together the yogurt, honey, juice of ½ lime and matcha green tea powder.

Evenly fill four martini glasses with the yogurt mixture. Top with the kiwi balls and garnish each with the lime zest, shaved coconut and a sprig of mint.

PER SERVING: Calories: 214, Fat: 8.8g, Protein: 6.4g, Sodium: 25mg, Fiber: 5.8g, Carbohydrates: 34g, Sugar: 22g

VERY BERRY PROTEIN PANCAKES

Protein powder gives this usually carb-heavy breakfast an extra-filling boost, helping you stay focused all morning.

INGREDIENTS

DIRECTIONS

SERVES 2–4

- 4 **eggs, separated**
- 4 **scoops vanilla-flavored vegan protein powder**
- 2 **teaspoons baking powder**
- 1 **tablespoon olive oil**
- 2 **cups mixed berries**
- 4 **sprigs of mint for garnish**

Whisk the egg whites with a hand or electric mixer until soft peaks form.

Mix the protein powder, egg yolks and baking powder together in a medium bowl. Fold the egg whites into batter.

Heat a pan or griddle over medium heat, coat with oil and add ¼ cup pancake batter. Cook the pancakes until bubbles stop forming on the top of the batter. Turn and continue to cook until the bottom is golden brown. Continue until all of the batter has been used.

Serve the pancakes with berries and a sprig of mint.

PER SERVING: Calories: 231, Fat: 8.4g, Protein: 24g, Sodium: 365mg, Fiber: 5.5g, Carbohydrates: 13g, Sugar: 5.9g

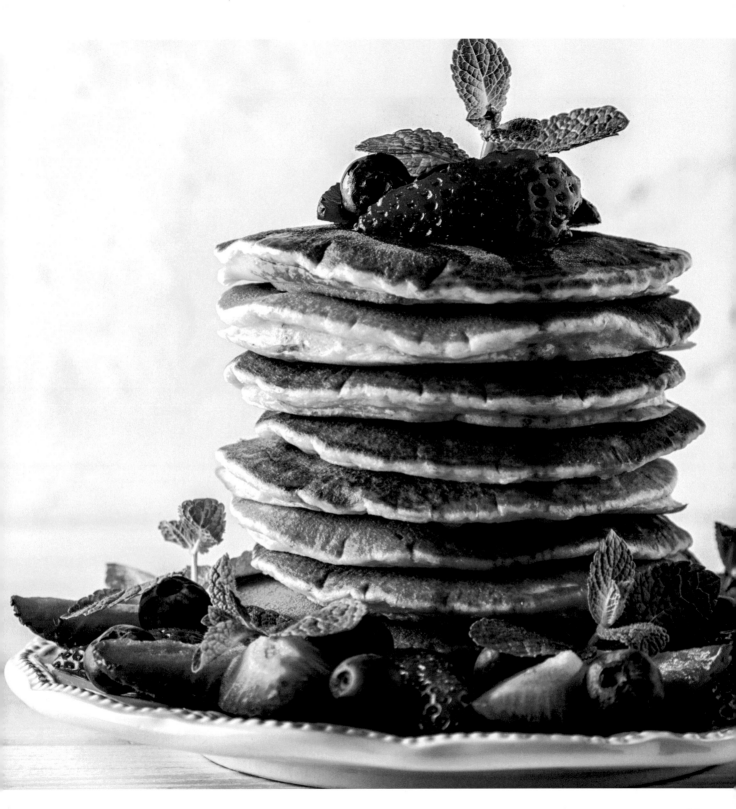

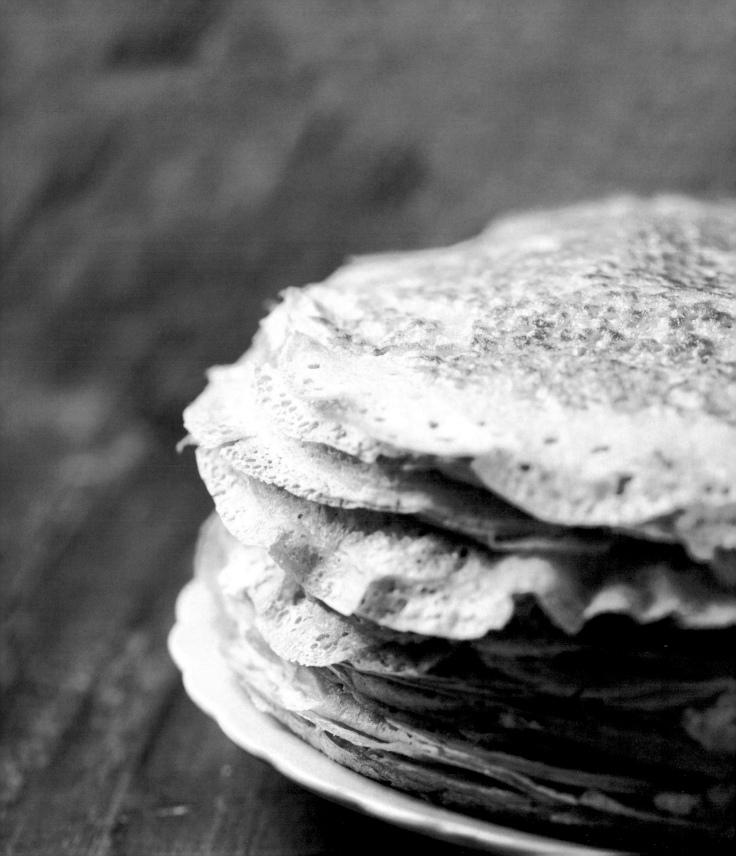

CRAB CREPES

These crepes are stuffed with crab and served with hollandaise sauce—they would be the star of a showstopper brunch.

| INGREDIENTS | DIRECTIONS | SERVES 4 |

INGREDIENTS

CREPES

- ½ cup millet flour
- ½ cup brown rice flour
- 1¼ cups unsweetened almond milk
- 1 avocado
- 1 tablespoon maple syrup
- Pinch fine sea salt
- Butter, for greasing pan

HOLLANDAISE SAUCE

- 2 large egg yolks
- 1 tablespoon lemon juice
- ½ teaspoon sea salt
- ½ cup butter, melted

FILLING

- 3 cups lump wild crab meat

DIRECTIONS

In a blender, add all crepe ingredients except the butter and blend until smooth.

Heat a nonstick pan over medium heat and coat with butter. Place a thin coating of crepe batter (about ¼ cup) into the pan, swirling it to distribute the batter as evenly as possible. Cook for about 1 minute, or until batter starts to bubble. Flip and cook another minute. Remove from pan and set aside. Continue in the same manner, greasing the pan for each crepe, until the batter is gone. Place parchment paper between crepes.

In a blender, add all hollandaise sauce ingredients except butter. Blend until thickened. While still blending, stream in the melted butter until the sauce is thick and creamy. Add water if the sauce becomes too thick.

Evenly distribute the crab among the crepes. Fold over, then fold in half. Drizzle each with hollandaise sauce and serve.

PER SERVING: Calories: 591, Fat: 36g, Protein: 35g, Sodium: 1,505mg, Fiber: 6g, Carbohydrates: 37g, Sugar: 7g

SAUSAGE BREAKFAST FRITTATA

Blending the eggs in this recipe might seem like an unnecessary step, but it's a great way to incorporate a lot of air and make a light and fluffy frittata!

INGREDIENTS

- 1 large breakfast sausage link
- 1 tablespoon butter
- ½ pound cremini mushrooms, cleaned and sliced
- 2 cups spinach
- 12 large eggs
- ½ teaspoon sea salt
- ½ teaspoon freshly ground black pepper
- 3 ounces goat cheese, crumbled
- Parsley for garnish (optional)

DIRECTIONS

SERVES 4-6

Preheat oven to 350 degrees F.

In a large cast-iron skillet coated with butter, cook the sausage until browned on all sides and cooked through. Set aside.

In the same skillet, cook the mushrooms until slightly brown and softened. Add in spinach and continue to cook until the spinach is wilted.

Add the eggs, salt and pepper into a blender and blend until the eggs are just blended.

Add the sausage back into the skillet. Add cheese and eggs into the skillet, transfer to the oven and cook for 20 to 30 minutes. Do not overcook.

Take out of the oven, garnish with parsely if desired and serve.

PER SERVING: Calories: 337, Fat: 26g, Protein: 21g, Sodium: 626mg, Fiber: 0.4g, Carbohydrates: 3.5g, Sugar: 1.6g

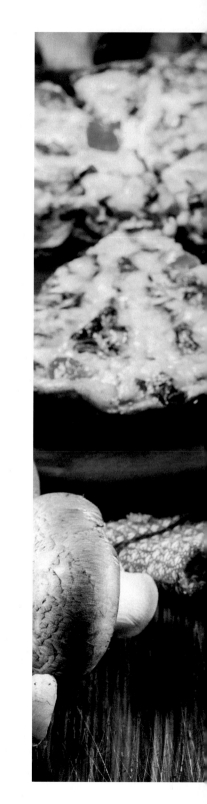

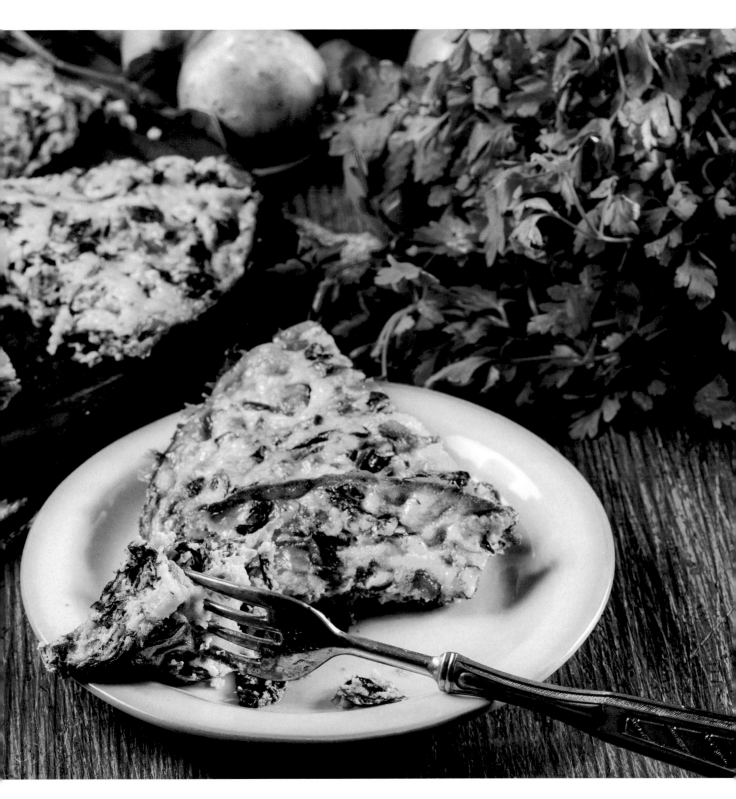

BREAKFAST SALMON SCRAMBLE

Use up your leftover salmon in this impossibly easy and delicious breakfast scramble.

INGREDIENTS

1 tablespoon butter

8 eggs

¼ teaspoon sea salt

¼ teaspoon freshly ground black pepper

8 ounces canned or cooked wild salmon, cut into bite-size pieces

2 cups fresh baby spinach

1 cup grape tomatoes, sliced

¼ cup fresh chives, chopped, plus extra for garnish

¼ cup Avocado Crema (page 163)

DIRECTIONS

SERVES 2-4

In a blender or large bowl, mix together the eggs.

In a large nonstick frying pan coated with butter, cook the eggs until they are almost done, stirring often. Season the eggs with salt and pepper.

Fold in the salmon, spinach, tomatoes and chives. Continue to cook until the eggs are just done and still slightly wet, stirring carefully to not break the salmon. Place the cooked eggs on a serving dish. Drizzle with the Avocado Crema and garnish with more chives.

PER SERVING: Calories: 154, Fat: 8.6g, Protein: 16g, Sodium: 571mg, Fiber: 2.5g, Carbohydrates: 4.8g, Sugar: 0.8g

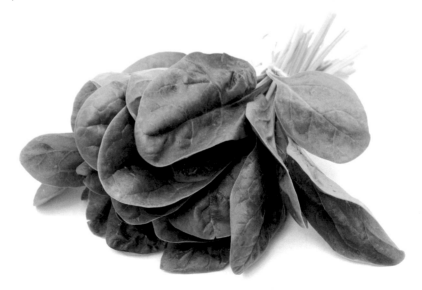

EGGS AND GARDEN VEGETABLE SPREAD

This Garden Vegetable Spread is ideal for using up a lot of leftover vegetables. It goes wonderfully with eggs, but it can also be used as a sandwich spread, in salad dressings or as a crust for chicken. The options are endless!

INGREDIENTS	DIRECTIONS	SERVES 4

GARDEN VEGETABLE SPREAD

- 1 large eggplant, peeled, seeded and chopped
- 1 large squash, peeled, seeded and chopped
- 7–10 ripe tomatoes, peeled, seeded and chopped
- 1 large onion, diced
- 2 stalks celery, diced
- 3 large carrots, diced
- 3 cloves garlic, peeled
- 3 tablespoons olive oil
- 1 tablespoon salt
- 1 tablespoon freshly ground black pepper
- 1 cup fresh kale or spinach
- ¼ cup fresh basil
- Small bunch parsley
- Vegetable broth, if needed

EGGS

- 8 eggs
- Fresh basil, for garnish

Preheat oven to 350 degrees F.

On a sheet pan lined with parchment paper, place the eggplant, squash, tomatoes, onion, celery, carrots and garlic. Drizzle with olive oil and season with salt and pepper. Mix the vegetables to coat evenly. Place in the oven and cook until vegetables are tender, about 35 minutes. Take out of oven and let cool.

Once cooled, place all vegetables and herbs in a food processor or blender and blend (you may have to do this in batches) until they have a smooth and spreadable consistency. If the sauce is too thick, add vegetable broth. Season to taste with salt and pepper.

Place 4 cups Garden Vegetable Spread into an oven-safe skillet. Warm the sauce on medium heat, stirring often. Set the oven to broil. Crack the eggs on top of the spread and place in the oven on the middle rack. Cook until the egg whites are set but the yolks are still runny, about 4 minutes. Remove from the oven and garnish with fresh basil.

PER SERVING: Calories: 390, Fat: 21g, Protein: 19g, Sodium: 1,558mg, Fiber: 11g, Carbohydrates: 33g, Sugar: 20g

GRANOLA BARS

These granola bars make for great grab-and-go breakfasts. Store leftovers in the freezer and let them defrost whenever you need a snack!

INGREDIENTS

DIRECTIONS

- ½ cup almonds
- ½ cup pistachios
- ½ cup walnuts
- ½ cup macadamias
- ¾ cup dark chocolate chips, 80% cocoa
- 1 cup shaved unsweetened coconut
- ¼ cup honey
- 1 tablespoon coconut sugar

In a bowl, mix together the nuts, chocolate and coconut.

In a small saucepan on medium-low heat, warm up the honey and sugar together until the sugar has melted. Add the honey mixture to the bowl and stir to coat all ingredients. Transfer to an 8" × 8" parchment-lined pan and press ingredients down tightly, making an even thickness. Cover with another piece of parchment paper and press against the mixture again. Place in the refrigerator to set for at least 2 hours.

Once set, remove from the refrigerator and cut into desired-size bars.

Note: Store leftover cut granola bars in the refrigerator or freezer.

PER SERVING: Calories: 737, Fat: 59g, Protein: 12g, Sodium: 10mg, Fiber: 9.8g, Carbohydrates: 57g, Sugar: 41g

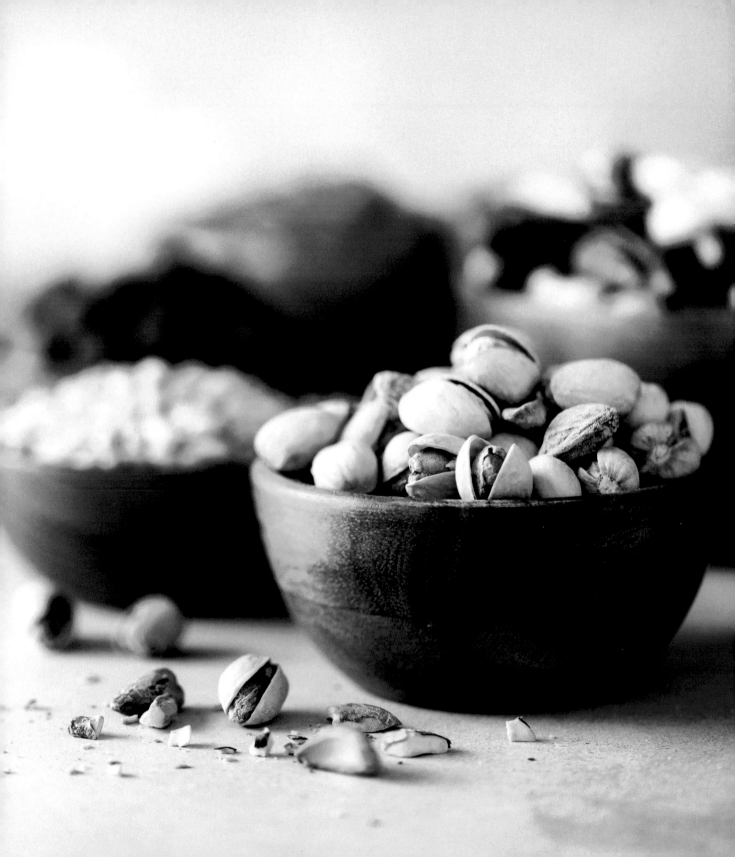

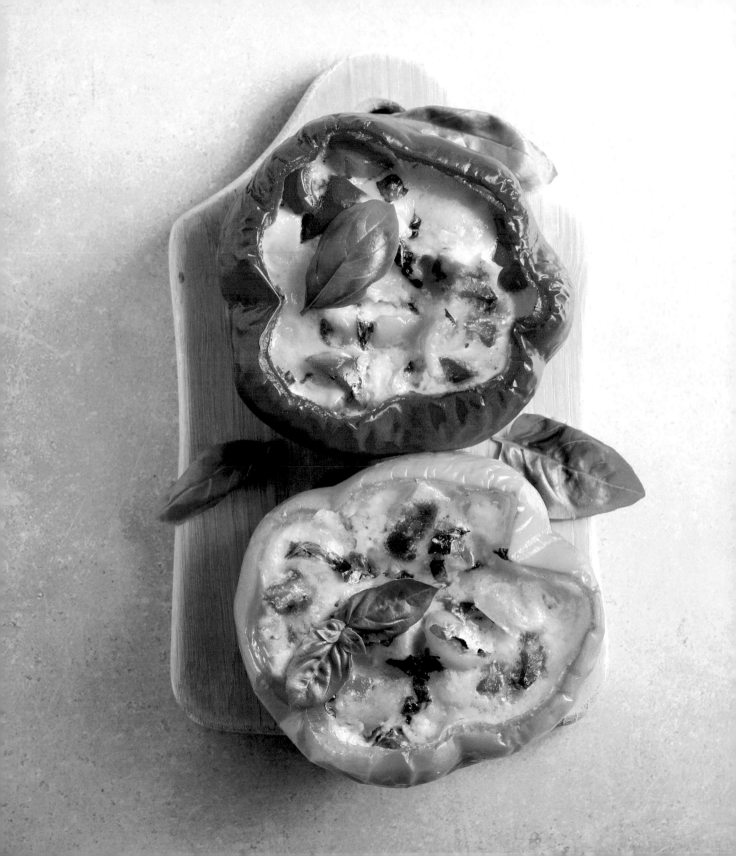

OMELET-STUFFED PEPPERS

You can use any bell peppers for this recipe, but using a combination
of colors makes for an extra-pleasing presentation.

INGREDIENTS

- 4 bell peppers
- 8 eggs
- ½ cup almond milk
- 1 teaspoon sea salt
- 1 teaspoon freshly ground black pepper
- 4 slices bacon, cooked and chopped
- 1 small onion, diced
- ½ cup red pepper, diced
- 3 ounces goat cheese
- 2 tablespoons sun-dried tomatoes, minced
- ¼ cup chives, chopped

DIRECTIONS

SERVES 4

Preheat oven to 375 degrees F.

Wash and dry the peppers. Cut off the tops and scoop out the seeds.

In a medium bowl mix together the eggs, milk, salt and pepper.

In another medium bowl, mix together all other ingredients. Evenly place the vegetable mixture into each pepper. Pour in the egg mixture and place the peppers in an oven-safe baking dish.

Cook in preheated oven for 15 to 20 minutes, or until the eggs are cooked and the pepper is soft.

PER SERVING: Calories: 334, Fat: 19g, Protein: 22g, Sodium: 823mg, Fiber: 3.5g, Carbohydrates: 19g, Sugar: 4.2g

ORANGE POMEGRANATE CREPES

These fruit-filled crepes are a surprisingly light and tasty way to start your day!

INGREDIENTS

CREPES

- ½ cup millet flour
- ½ cup brown rice flour
- 1¼ cups unsweetened almond milk
- 1 organic avocado
- 1 tablespoon organic maple syrup
- Pinch fine sea salt
- Butter

FILLING

- 3 organic oranges
- ¼ cup organic maple syrup
- ¼ teaspoon sea salt
- 1 pomegranate
- Mint for garnish

DIRECTIONS

SERVES 4

In a blender, add all crepe ingredients except the butter and blend until smooth.

Heat a nonstick pan over medium heat and coat with butter. Place a thin coating of crepe batter (about ¼ cup) into the pan, swirling it to distribute the batter as evenly as possible. Cook for about 1 minute or until the batter starts to bubble. Flip and cook another minute. Remove from pan and set aside. Continue in the same manner, greasing the pan for each crepe, until the batter is gone. Place parchment paper between each cooked crepe.

Zest 1 orange and set aside zest. Peel the skin and pith (white part) from this orange as well as a second orange. Then, over a bowl to catch the orange juice, segment both oranges by cutting between the segments. Reserve the juice.

In a small pot over medium-low heat, add in the reserved orange juice, the reserved zest, maple syrup, and salt. Bring to a simmer and cook until sauce reduces and thickens, about 3 to 5 minutes. Add orange segments to the filling.

Slice the last orange into rounds.

Fill crepes with orange filling and fold over, then fold in half. Peel half the skin off the pomegranate and tap the unpeeled side with a wooden spoon to release pomegranate seeds.

Place desired amount of pomegranate seeds onto crepes and garnish with orange rounds and mint.

PER SERVING: Calories: 385, Fat: 11g, Protein: 6.6g, Sodium: 45mg, Fiber: 9.8g, Carbohydrates: 69g, Sugar: 34g

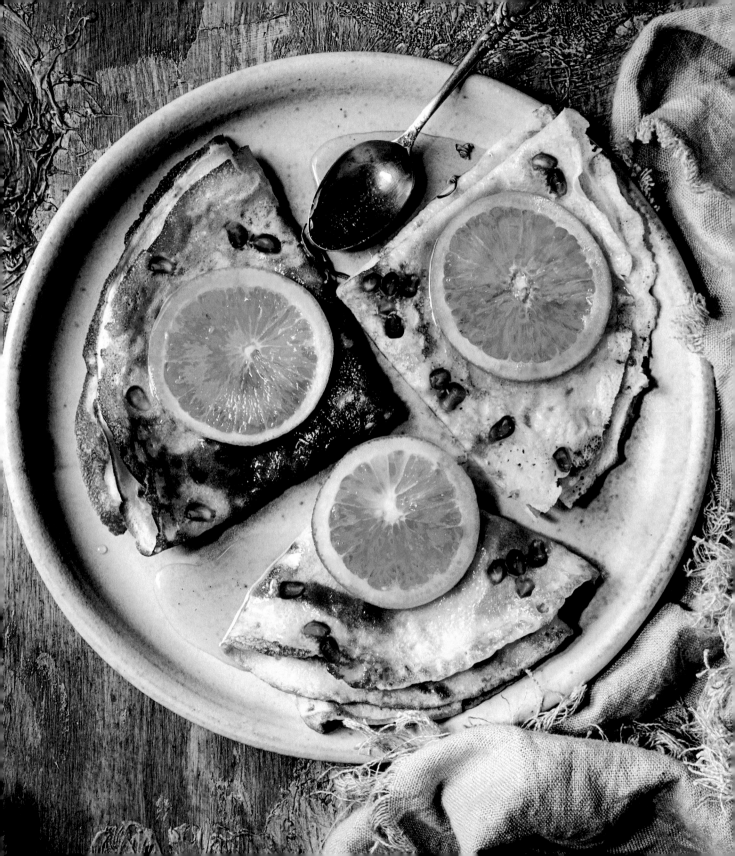

SWEET POTATO AND PULLED PORK EGGS BENEDICT

This Southwest-inspired variation on eggs Benedict is a great choice when you need something a little different to start your day.

INGREDIENTS

DIRECTIONS

SERVES 4

SWEET POTATO CAKES

- 2 sweet potatoes, shredded
- 2 tablespoons olive oil
- 1 small onion
- ½ red bell pepper
- 1 clove garlic, minced
- 2 eggs
- ½ teaspoon sea salt
- ½ teaspoon freshly ground black pepper
- Oil for frying (olive or avocado)

CHILI LIME HOLLANDAISE SAUCE

- 2 large egg yolks
- 1 tablespoon lime juice
- ½ teaspoon sea salt
- 1 teaspoon chili powder
- ½ cup butter, melted

TOPPING

- 4 eggs
- Pulled Pork (page 172)
- Apple Slaw (page 132)
- Avocado Crema (page 163)

In a large bowl, combine the shredded sweet potatoes and 1 tablespoon oil, mixing to coat the potatoes with oil. Place in a microwave oven for 2 to 3 minutes, or until potatoes are softened, mixing halfway through. Set aside to cool.

Heat a small pan coated with 1 tablespoon oil over medium heat. Cook the onions and peppers until soft, about 2 to 4 minutes. Add in the garlic and cook for another minute. Let cool.

In a small bowl, beat the eggs together.

Add the vegetable mixture and eggs to the sweet potatoes. Season with salt and pepper and mix together. Form the mixture into four patties.

Heat ¾ inch oil in a large nonstick frying pan. Fry the sweet potato patties on both sides until browned and crispy. Drain on paper towels.

In a blender, add all hollandaise sauce ingredients except the butter and blend until thickened. While still blending, stream in the melted butter until sauce is thick and creamy. Add water if it becomes too thick.

Bring a large pan of water to a gentle boil. Crack eggs one at a time into a small fine mesh sieve and let the runny whites run out of the sieve. Stir with a spoon to make a swirl in the water. Carefully place the eggs into the water and cook for 2 to 3 minutes. Scoop the eggs from the water with a slotted spoon and drain on paper towels.

Place sweet potato cakes on serving plates, top each with the desired amount of Pulled Pork, a little spoonful of Apple Slaw, a poached egg and spoon over a good amount of chili lime hollandaise sauce, then a drizzle of Avocado Crema on top of the hollandaise.

PER SERVING: Calories: 1,186, Fat: 82g, Protein: 43g, Sodium: 2,121mg, Fiber: 12g, Carbohydrates: 70g, Sugar: 43g

START-YOUR-DAY SMOOTHIE BOWL

This smoothie bowl is chock-full of good-for-you ingredients, helping you start the day right.

INGREDIENTS

- 2 cups kombucha
- 2 sliced beets
- 1 large kale leaf, stem removed
- 1 teaspoon matcha green tea powder
- 1 cup ice
- 1 lemon, juiced
- 1 cup blueberries, plus extra for garnish
- 2 tablespoons chia seeds
- Coconut flakes
- ¼ cup pomegranate seeds

DIRECTIONS

In a blender, add the kombucha, beets, kale, lemon juice, matcha, blueberries and ice. Blend until smooth, adding more kombucha if needed.

Pour into two bowls. Mix 1 tablespoon chia seeds into each bowl. Top each bowl evenly with coconut flakes, blueberries and pomegranate seeds.

PER SERVING: Calories: 221, Fat: 6.9g, Protein: 7.9g, Sodium: 77mg, Fiber: 12g, Carbohydrates: 42g, Sugar: 26g

SERVES 2

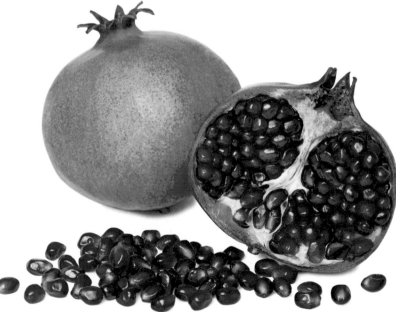

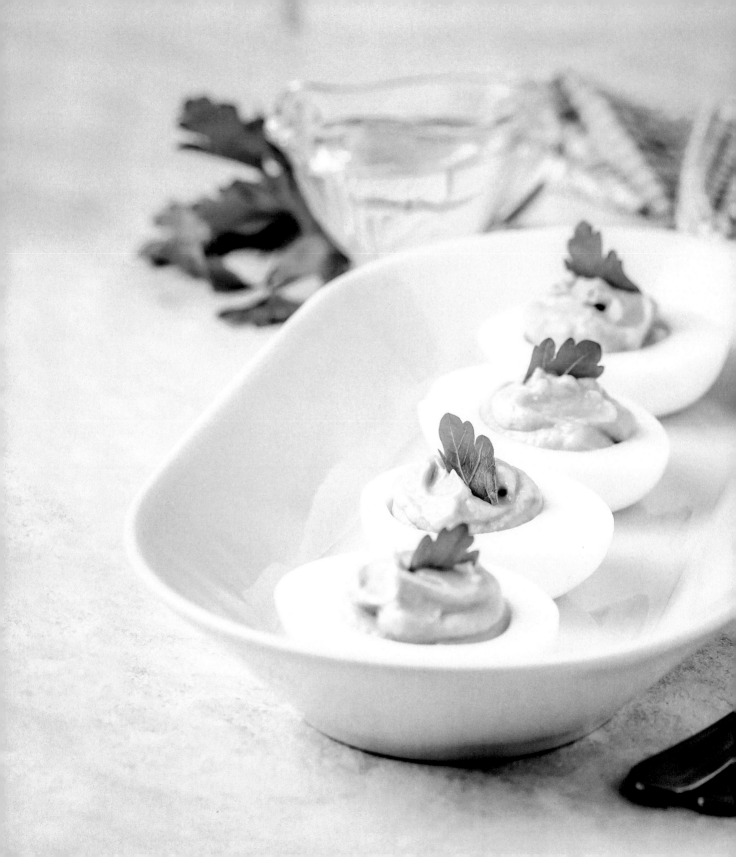

snacks & starters

THESE SMALL BITES ARE PERFECT FOR ENTERTAINING.

Rustic Grilled Peach Bruschetta 66

Black Rice Cakes with Scallops and Leek Cream Sauce 68

Mini Sliders with Brussels Sprout Buns 69

Salmon Salad Appetizers 70

Roasted Eggplants 70

Spicy Coconut Shrimp with Pegan Cocktail Sauce 73

Vegetable-Stuffed Tomatoes 74

Grilled Zucchini and Tomato Roll-Ups 74

Dukkah Kale Chips 75

Guacamole Deviled Eggs 76

Grilled Green Oysters 78

Beet Chip Nachos with Refried Lentils 81

Sweet Potato Toast 82

Beef-Wrapped Vegetable Bundles 83

Spaghetti Squash Cakes 84

Vegetable and Shrimp Ceviche 87

Stuffed Sweet Potato Snacks 89

Steamed Chicken and Vegetable Pinwheels 90

Vegetable-Stuffed Artichokes 91

Fried Anchovies 93

RUSTIC GRILLED PEACH BRUSCHETTA

This grilled fruit appetizer is naturally sweet—you might prefer having it for dessert!

INGREDIENTS

- 4 large peaches
- 1 tablespoon olive oil
- ½ cup sheep's milk feta
- 5 basil leaves
- ¼ cup balsamic drizzle

DIRECTIONS

SERVES 4

Preheat the grill to medium-high.

Cut the peaches in half, take the pits out and place peaches on a hot, oiled grill.

Cook just a couple of minutes, or until peaches have grill marks and are just softened. Cut each peach half into four slices and place on a serving plate.

Stack the basil leaves, roll them tightly and slice the leaves perpendicular to the roll to make thin strips.

Crumble the feta over the peaches. Drizzle with balsamic and top with basil. Serve with your favorite pegan crackers.

PER SERVING: Calories: 178, Fat: 9.7g, Protein: 6g, Sodium: 326mg, Fiber: 2.4g, Carbohydrates: 18g, Sugar: 16g

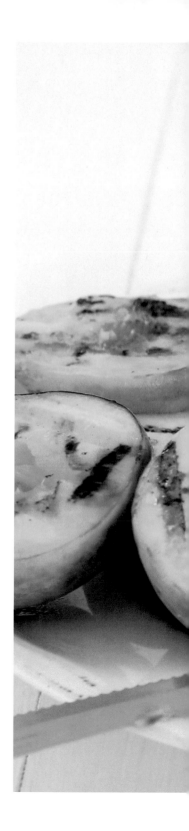

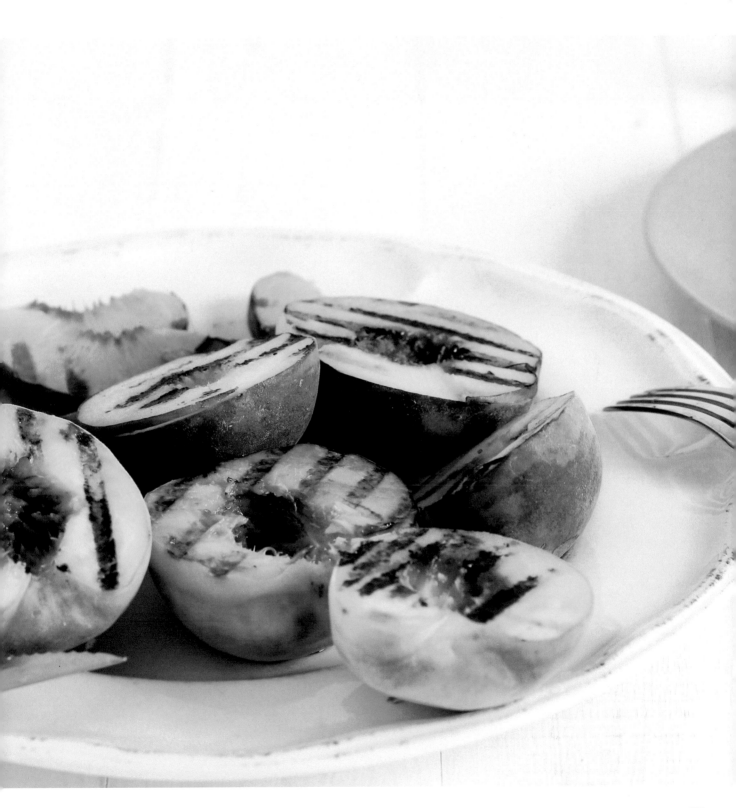

BLACK RICE CAKES WITH SCALLOPS AND LEEK CREAM SAUCE

If you're looking for an impressive appetizer, look no further.
These rice cakes and scallops would fit in at any black-tie affair.

INGREDIENTS

RICE CAKES

- 1 cup uncooked black rice
- 1¾ cups water
- 2 eggs, whisked
- 1 tablespoon fresh chives
- ¼ cup ripe tomato, seeded and diced
- 2 cloves garlic, minced
- ½ teaspoon sea salt
- ½ teaspoon freshly ground black pepper
- 2 tablespoons fresh parsley, finely chopped
- 3 tablespoons olive oil

LEEK CREAM SAUCE

- 1 cup leeks, cleaned and thinly sliced
- 1 tablespoon butter
- 1 clove garlic, minced
- ¼ cup vegetable broth
- ¼ teaspoon sea salt
- ¼ teaspoon freshly ground black pepper
- ¼ cup coconut cream

SCALLOPS

- 1 pound scallops
- ½ teaspoon sea salt
- ¼ teaspoon freshly ground black pepper
- 1 tablespoon butter

DIRECTIONS

Add water and rice to a small saucepan. Bring to a boil, reduce heat and simmer covered for 30 minutes, or until the rice is tender and most of the water has absorbed. Let cool.

In a medium bowl, mix together the cooked, cooled rice and the remaining rice cake ingredients except for the oil.

Make 2-inch cakes from the rice mixture and fry in a large nonstick pan with oil over medium heat until crisp and browned on both sides, about 2 to 3 minutes per side. Drain on paper towels.

Heat a medium saucepan over medium. Add butter and cook the leeks for a couple of minutes. Add in garlic and cook for another minute. Stir in broth, salt and pepper and simmer to reduce liquid by ¼. Stir in cream and simmer for a couple more minutes to thicken.

Season scallops with salt and pepper. Heat a medium nonstick pan on medium-high and add butter. Sear scallops for a couple of minutes on each side, or until scallops are no longer opaque.

Place rice cakes on a serving platter. Top each with a scallop, drizzle with leek cream sauce and serve.

PER SERVING: Calories: 239, Fat: 16g, Protein: 13g, Sodium: 698mg, Fiber: 0.8g, Carbohydrates: 12g, Sugar: 1.6g

MINI SLIDERS WITH BRUSSELS SPROUT BUNS

Roasted Brussels sprouts make for adorable buns in these tiny and tempting sliders.

| INGREDIENTS | DIRECTIONS | SERVES 4 |

INGREDIENTS

SPROUTS

16–20 Brussels sprouts, halved

1 tablespoon olive oil

½ teaspoon sea salt

½ teaspoon freshly ground black pepper

TOPPINGS

1 tablespoon olive oil

1 large onion, thinly sliced

¼ teaspoon sea salt

BURGERS

1¼ pounds 80/20 ground beef

2 tablespoons store-bought hamburger seasoning, or your own blend

DIRECTIONS

Preheat oven to 375 degrees F.

On a parchment-lined sheet pan, place the Brussels sprouts, oil, salt and pepper. Mix to coat evenly. Arrange each sprout cut-side down. Place in preheated oven and cook for 15 to 20 minutes, or until fork-tender.

In a nonstick pan with oil on medium heat, add onions and salt and cook for about 10 minutes, or until the onions are soft and caramelized, stirring frequently.

Combine the ground beef with seasoning. Form into as many mini patties as you have Brussels sprout "buns." Grill the burgers in a cast-iron or nonstick pan until cooked through, about 2 minutes on each side.

Take the Brussels sprouts out of the oven, turn half of them over and place a mini burger on top of each. Top each with some caramelized onion and the other sprout half. Spear with a toothpick to secure.

PER SERVING: Calories: 485, Fat: 35g, Protein: 28g, Sodium: 562mg, Fiber: 4.6g, Carbohydrates: 15g, Sugar: 3.8g

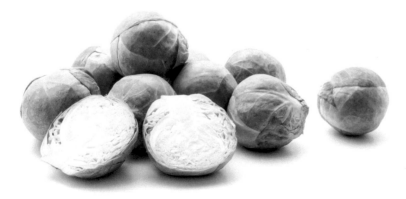

SALMON SALAD APPETIZERS

Salmon, dill and cucumber are a classic combination for a reason!
These light, refreshing and crunchy bites are a guaranteed crowd-pleaser.

INGREDIENTS
DIRECTIONS
SERVES 4-6

- 4 ounces wild salmon, cooked
- ½ cup sheep's yogurt
- 1 tablespoon dill, finely chopped, plus extra for garnish
- ½ lemon zest
- ¼ teaspoon sea salt
- ¼ teaspoon freshly ground black pepper
- 1 English cucumber, sliced in ¼-inch rounds

Break up the salmon into smaller-than-bite-size pieces.

In a medium bowl, mix together the salmon, yogurt, dill, lemon zest, salt and pepper.

Place a dollop of salmon salad onto the sliced cucumbers and garnish with a small dill sprig.

PER SERVING: Calories: 72, Fat: 3.2g, Protein: 8.6g, Sodium: 233mg, Fiber: 0.3g, Carbohydrates: 3.2g, Sugar: 1.4g

ROASTED EGGPLANTS

This rustic eggplant appetizer becomes an excellent topping for pegan crackers after roasting in the oven with garlic, red pepper and thyme.

INGREDIENTS
DIRECTIONS
SERVES 4-6

- 6 baby eggplants
- 2 tablespoons olive oil
- 3 cloves garlic, minced
- ¼ teaspoon red pepper flakes
- ½ tablespoon fresh thyme
- ¼ teaspoon sea salt
- ¼ teaspoon freshly ground black pepper
- 1 lemon

Preheat oven to 350 degrees F.

Wash and cut each eggplant lengthwise into ¼-inch-thick slices.

Place the eggplant slices on a parchment-lined cookie sheet. Drizzle the slices with olive oil and evenly top with garlic, red pepper, thyme, salt and pepper. Bake the eggplant in a preheated oven for 20 minutes, or until tender.

Place the roasted eggplant on a serving platter. Cut the lemon in half and squeeze the juice over the roasted eggplant. Serve the remaining lemon half on the side. Enjoy with your favorite pegan crackers.

PER SERVING: Calories: 126, Fat: 6.8g, Protein: 3g, Sodium: 110mg, Fiber: 6g, Carbohydrates: 17g, Sugar: 6.3g

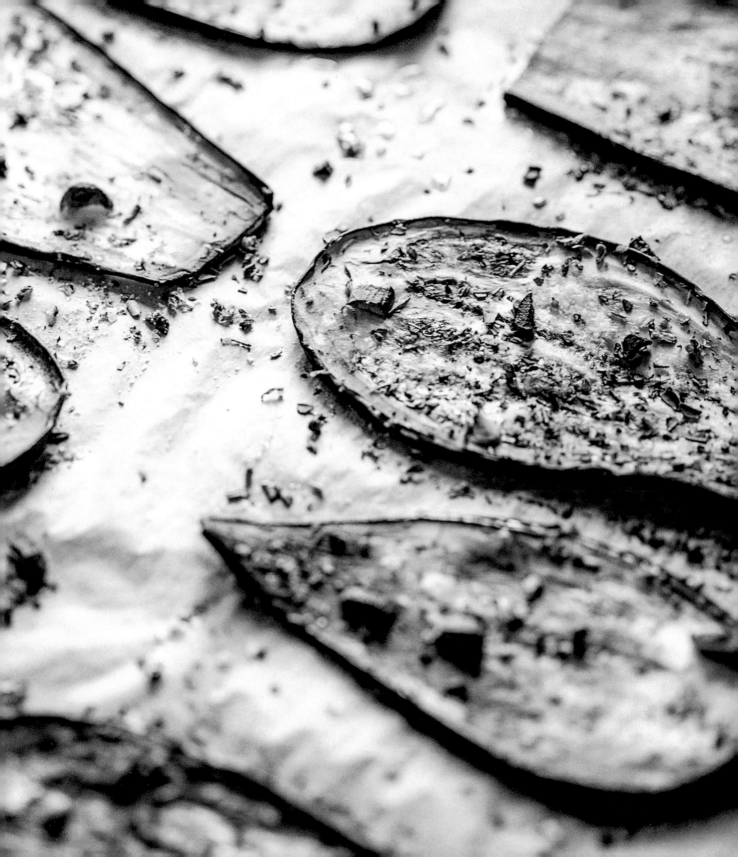

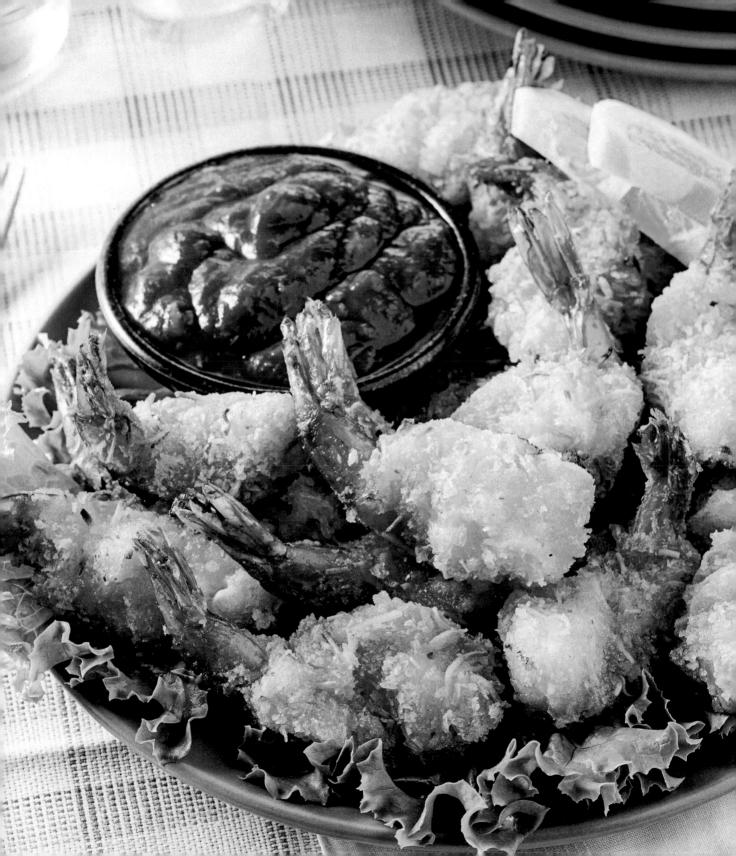

SPICY COCONUT SHRIMP WITH PEGAN COCKTAIL SAUCE

If a whole minced chili sounds like too much spice for you, start with ⅛ teaspoon cayenne powder instead.

PEGAN KETCHUP

- 5 ripe tomatoes, chopped
- 1 sweet onion, chopped
- 1 tablespoon olive oil
- 2 cloves garlic, minced
- 2 tablespoons balsamic vinegar
- 2 tablespoons fresh basil, minced
- 2 tablespoons fresh parsley, minced

PEGAN COCKTAIL SAUCE

- 1 cup Pegan Ketchup
- 2 tablespoons horseradish

SPICY COCONUT SHRIMP

- 1 cup unsweetened coconut flour
- 3 eggs
- ½ cup unsweetened shredded coconut
- 2 tablespoons minced green onion
- 1 hot chili pepper, minced, some seeds removed
- 1 pound (21–25) tail-on jumbo shrimp, shelled and deveined
- Oil for deep frying

KETCHUP & COCKTAIL SAUCE

Preheat oven to 350 degrees F.

Place tomatoes and onions on a parchment-lined cookie sheet. Drizzle the vegetables with oil and mix to coat. Cook 10 to 15 minutes, or until the vegetables are soft. Add garlic to the pan and cook another minute.

Heat a medium saucepan on medium-low heat. Add the roasted vegetables and remaining ketchup ingredients. Simmer sauce for 10 to 15 minutes, or until reduced by ¼. Remove from heat and cool. Pegan Ketchup will keep in an airtight container in the refrigerator for 10 days.

Mix 1 cup pegan ketchup with 2 tablespoons horseradish to make Pegan Cocktail Sauce.

SPICY COCONUT SHRIMP

Set up a coating station with three separate shallow bowls. In the first bowl, add the coconut flour. In the second bowl, beat the eggs together. In the third bowl, combine the shredded coconut, onion and chili pepper.

Coat each shrimp with flour, then cover with egg and coat with the coconut mixture. Set aside the prepared shrimp on a plate.

Heat a deep fryer or wide saucepan with 1 to 2 inches of oil. Heat oil to 360 degrees F and add the shrimp in small batches until golden brown, about 3 to 4 minutes. Drain on paper towels.

Serve with the Pegan Cocktail Sauce.

PER SERVING: Calories: 569, Fat: 22g, Protein: 40g, Sodium: 1,524mg, Fiber: 15g, Carbohydrates: 51g, Sugar: 29g

VEGETABLE-STUFFED TOMATOES

Sometimes easy appetizers are the tastiest. This one comes together in a snap, especially if you have leftover Vegetable Chop and Avocado Crema in your refrigerator.

INGREDIENTS	DIRECTIONS	SERVES 4

INGREDIENTS

16 ripe grape tomatoes

1½ cups Vegetable Chop (page 146)

Drizzle of Avocado Crema (page 163)

DIRECTIONS

Wash and dry the tomatoes. Cut off the tops and use a small spoon to scoop out the pulp. Fill each with Vegetable Chop, drizzle with Avocado Crema and serve.

PER SERVING: Calories: 90, Fat: 5.3g, Protein: 3.2g, Sodium: 142mg, Fiber: 2.9g, Carbohydrates: 9g, Sugar: 2.6g

GRILLED ZUCCHINI AND TOMATO ROLL-UPS

Grilling the zucchini and tomatoes adds a touch of smoke to this light appetizer.

INGREDIENTS	DIRECTIONS	SERVES 4

INGREDIENTS

2 medium zucchinis

⅓ cup olive oil

½ teaspoon dried basil

½ teaspoon dried oregano

½ teaspoon dried parsley

½ teaspoon onion powder

½ teaspoon garlic powder

¼ teaspoon sea salt

¼ teaspoon freshly ground black pepper

1 pint ripe grape tomatoes

DIRECTIONS

Preheat grill to medium-high.

Using a mandolin, thinly slice the zucchini lengthwise into long strips.

In a wide, shallow bowl, mix together the oil, basil, oregano, parsley, onion powder, garlic powder, salt and pepper. Place cut zucchini into mixture to marinate for 10 minutes.

Place the zucchini and tomatoes on a preheated, well-greased grill and cook until the zucchini is pliable and the tomatoes are softened.

Roll the tomatoes with the zucchini and secure each with a toothpick. Place on a serving dish and drizzle with the remaining marinade.

PER SERVING: Calories: 195, Fat: 18g, Protein: 2.2g, Sodium: 14mg, Fiber: 2.2g, Carbohydrates: 7.6g, Sugar: 4.9g

DUKKAH KALE CHIPS

Dukkah spice makes these kale chips deliciously addictive!
If you're feeding a crowd, go ahead and make a double batch.

INGREDIENTS

- 1 large bunch fresh kale
- 1 tablespoon olive oil
- ½ teaspoon sea salt
- ½ teaspoon freshly ground black pepper
- 1 tablespoon dukkah, homemade (page 140) or store-bought

DIRECTIONS

SERVES 2–4

Preheat oven to 350 degrees F.

Wash and dry the kale. Remove the stems and tear the kale into chip-size pieces.

On a parchment-lined cookie sheet, place the kale, olive oil, salt, pepper and dukkah. Mix to coat evenly and spread out the kale so it overlaps as little as possible. Bake the kale in the preheated oven 10 to 15 minutes, or until the kale is crunchy. Add more salt and pepper if desired.

PER SERVING: Calories: 66, Fat: 4.7g, Protein: 2.6g, Sodium: 261mg, Fiber: 2g, Carbohydrates: 4.8g, Sugar: 1.1g

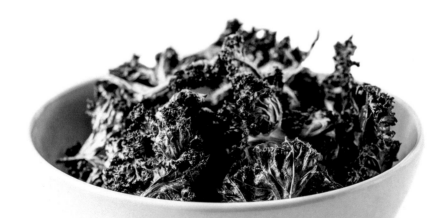

GUACAMOLE DEVILED EGGS

Avocado's healthy fats more than make up for the lack of mayonnaise in these Mexican-inspired deviled eggs.

| INGREDIENTS | DIRECTIONS | SERVES 4 |

INGREDIENTS

- 6 eggs
- 1 ripe avocado, peeled and pitted
- 1 tablespoon lime juice
- ¼ teaspoon sea salt
- ¼ teaspoon freshly ground black pepper
- 2 tablespoons red onion, finely diced
- ½ ripe tomato, finely diced
- 1 tablespoon jalapeño, seeded and finely diced
- 12 cilantro leaves
- 2 slices red cabbage (optional)

DIRECTIONS

Place the eggs in a saucepan and cover with cold water. Bring water to a boil over medium heat. Once the water has come to a boil, cover and remove it from heat. Let sit 12 minutes. Transfer the eggs to a bath of cold water.

Cut the eggs in half, scoop out the yolks and add them to a medium bowl. Add in the avocado, lime juice, salt and pepper. Smash the yolks and avocado with a fork and mix together until smooth.

In a small bowl, mix together the red onion, tomato and jalapeño.

Evenly pipe the avocado filling into the egg white halves. Top each with the tomato mixture and garnish with cilantro.

Optional: For purple eggs, add the hard-boiled eggs and cabbage to a saucepan and cover with water. Bring to a boil on high heat. Turn off the heat and let cool. Remove the cabbage from water. Crack the hard-boiled eggs a little on each side. Return them to the cabbage water and place it in the refrigerator until the desired color is reached. Remove the eggs from the water and peel.

PER SERVING: Calories: 190, Fat: 14g, Protein: 11g, Sodium: 220mg, Fiber: 3.3g, Carbohydrates: 6.1g, Sugar: 1.7g

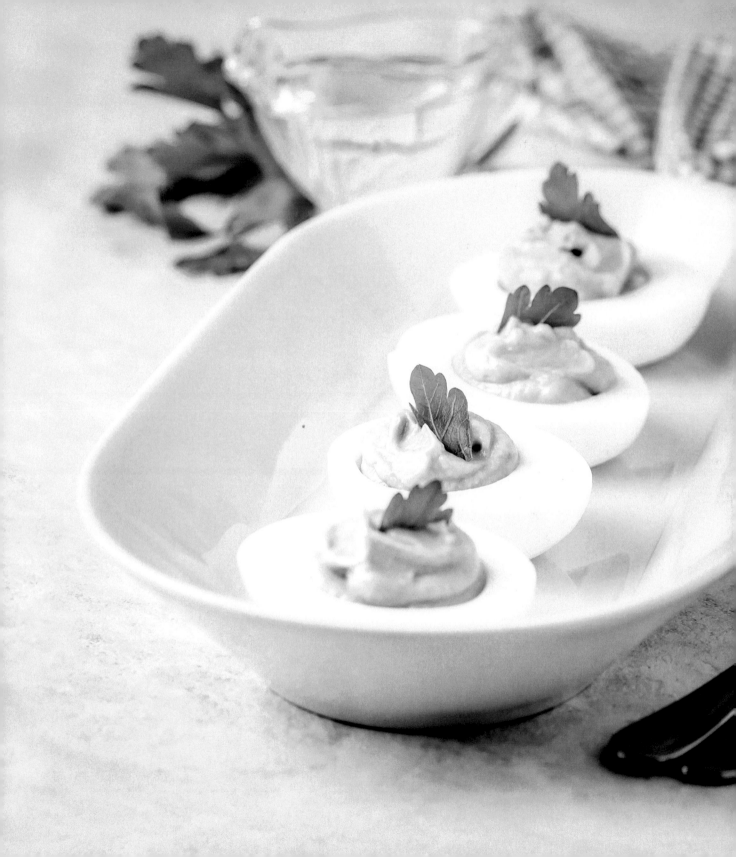

GRILLED GREEN OYSTERS

These summery, pesto-inspired oysters would make a special start to a dinner for two.

INGREDIENTS   **DIRECTIONS**   SERVES 1–2

- 4 tablespoons butter
- 1 cup baby spinach
- 2 tablespoons fresh parsley
- 2 cloves garlic
- ¼ teaspoon cayenne pepper
- ¼ teaspoon sea salt
- I dozen oysters on the half shell

Preheat grill on medium heat.

Melt the butter in a small saucepan or microwave.

Add the spinach, parsley, garlic, pepper and salt to a blender or food processor. Pulse ingredients together until broken down but not puréed.

Mix together the spinach mixture and melted butter. Evenly spoon the mixture onto the oysters.

Place the oysters on the preheated grill and cook for 4 minutes, or until the butter starts to sizzle in the shell and the oysters just start to cook. Remove from the grill and serve.

PER SERVING: Calories: 255, Fat: 25g, Protein: 5.8g, Sodium: 311mg, Fiber: 0.7g, Carbohydrates: 5g, Sugar: 0.5g

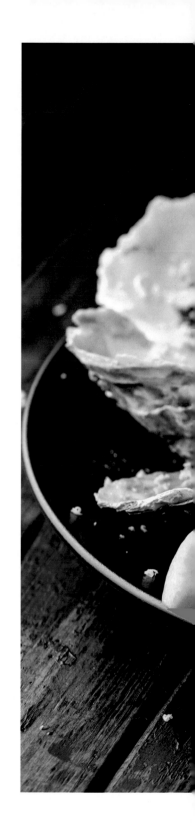

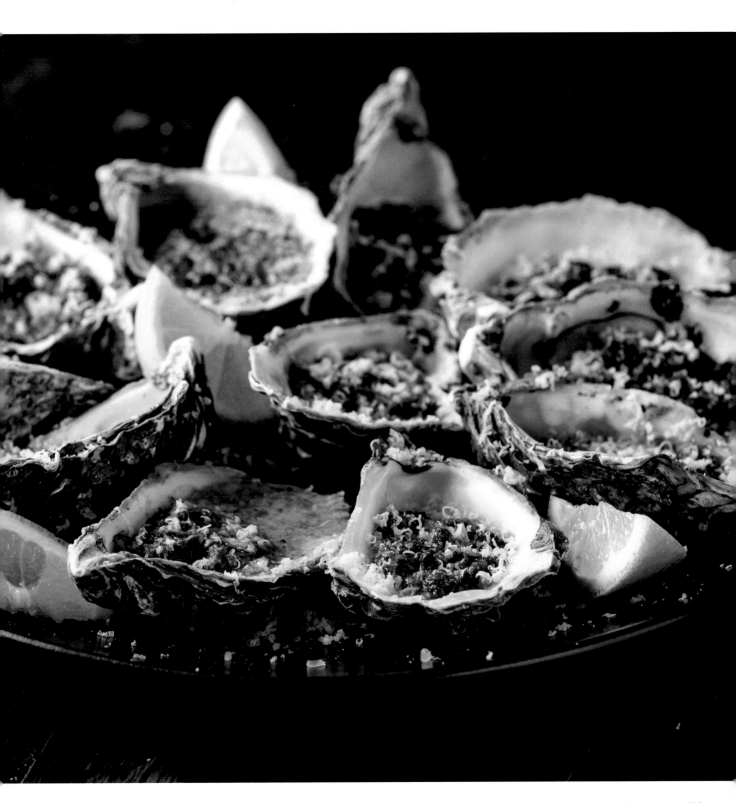

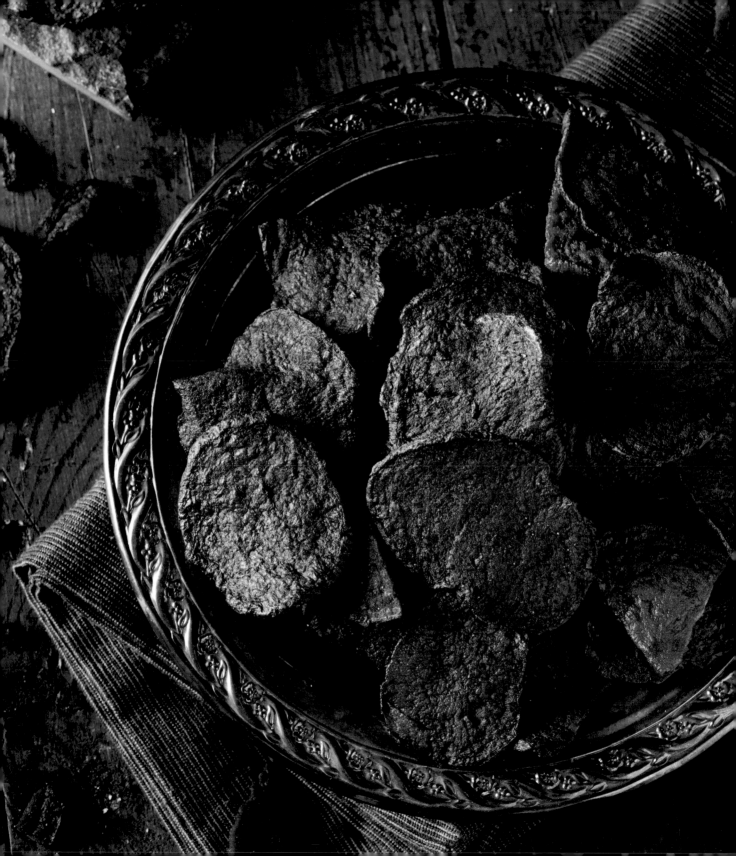

BEET CHIP NACHOS WITH REFRIED LENTILS

These colorful nachos are delicious and completely guilt-free!

| INGREDIENTS | DIRECTIONS | SERVES 4 |

INGREDIENTS

BEET CHIPS

- 3 beets, preferably in different colors
- 1 tablespoon olive oil
- ½ teaspoon sea salt
- ½ teaspoon pepper

REFRIED LENTILS

- 1 cup lentils
- 4 tablespoons olive oil
- 3 tablespoons red pepper, minced
- 2 tablespoons onion, minced
- 2 garlic cloves, minced
- ½ teaspoon cumin
- ½ teaspoon sea salt
- ½ teaspoon freshly ground black pepper

TOPPINGS

- ½ cup romaine lettuce, chopped
- 1 jalapeño, sliced
- ½ cup salsa
- 2 tablespoons chives, sliced
- Drizzle of Avocado Crema (page 163)

DIRECTIONS

Preheat oven to 350 degrees F.

Using a mandolin, thinly slice the beets. Line a cookie sheet with parchment paper and brush with olive oil. Place beets in a single layer onto cookie sheet and brush beets with remaining oil. Place in preheated oven and bake for 15 to 20 minutes. Remove from the oven and immediately season with salt and pepper.

Rinse lentils in cold water. Look for and remove any debris, then drain. Place lentils in a medium saucepan with enough water to cover lentils. Heat over medium-high heat and boil lentils until tender, about 15 to 20 minutes.

Heat a medium frying pan over medium. Coat with oil and cook the onion and pepper until soft, about 2 minutes. Add in garlic and cook another minute. Season with cumin, salt and pepper.

Drain the cooked lentils and add them to the frying pan. With a handheld potato masher, mash the lentils until half are broken up and mashed.

Arrange the beet chips on a serving platter and top with lentils, lettuce, jalapeño, salsa, chives and a generous drizzle of Avocado Crema.

PER SERVING: Calories: 370, Fat: 18g, Protein: 14g, Sodium: 643mg, Fiber: 19g, Carbohydrates: 40g, Sugar: 7g

SWEET POTATO TOAST

This recipe trades traditional grain toast for slices of sweet potato. It's a hearty snack designed to get you through that midafternoon slump.

INGREDIENTS

DIRECTIONS

SERVES 4

- 1 large sweet potato
- 2 tablespoons avocado oil
- 1 teaspoon salt
- 1 teaspoon freshly ground black pepper
- 4 eggs
- 1 cup Garden Vegetable Spread (page 55)
- 2 avocados, sliced
- 1 tablespoon dukkah, homemade (page 140) or store-bought
- ½ cup microgreens

Preheat oven to 350 degrees F.

Slice the sweet potatoes lengthwise, making four large, ⅓-inch-thick slices. Place the slices on a parchment-lined cookie sheet. Drizzle oil onto the potatoes and season with salt and pepper. Place in the oven and cook for 10 to 15 minutes, or until fork-tender.

Bring a saucepan of water to a boil over medium-high heat. Use a slotted spoon to carefully lower eggs into the boiling water. Lower heat to a simmer and cook the eggs for 6 minutes. Remove the eggs and place them in a bath of cold water for 2 minutes. Take the eggs from the water. Peel, slice and set aside.

Remove the potatoes from the oven. Place on serving plates, top each with Garden Vegetable Spread, sliced avocados, sliced eggs, dukkah and microgreens.

PER SERVING: Calories: 366, Fat: 29g, Protein: 9.9g, Sodium: 564mg, Fiber: 9.2g, Carbohydrates: 18g, Sugar: 2.1g

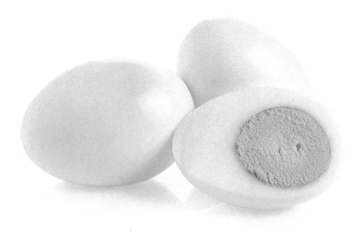

BEEF-WRAPPED VEGETABLE BUNDLES

These little bundles are the perfect beefy bite. The vegetable bundles and the balsamic glaze make for a winning flavor combination!

INGREDIENTS   DIRECTIONS   SERVES 4

STEAK

1½ pounds skirt steak

½ teaspoon sea salt

½ teaspoon freshly ground black pepper

VEGETABLE BUNDLES

2 carrots

1 red pepper

1 bunch asparagus tips

½ teaspoon sea salt

½ teaspoon freshly ground black pepper

2 tablespoon olive oil

BALSAMIC GLAZE

½ cup balsamic vinegar

1 sprig fresh thyme

1 clove garlic, minced

Preheat grill to medium-high.

Season the steak with salt and pepper. Place on a hot grill for 3 to 4 minutes per side, or until internal temperature reaches 135 degrees F. Let steak rest for 10 minutes before slicing.

Preheat oven to 350 degrees F.

Julienne carrots and peppers by slicing them into thin strips that resemble matchsticks.

Add the carrots, peppers and asparagus tips to a sheet pan lined with parchment paper. Toss with oil and season with salt and pepper. Roast for 10 to 15 minutes, or until the vegetables are fork-tender.

In a small saucepan over medium heat, add all balsamic glaze ingredients together and simmer for 3 to 4 minutes, or until thickened. Take out the thyme sprig.

If the steak is too long, cut in half, then slice against the grain of the steak.

Arrange the vegetables into little bundles with an even amount of each vegetable in each bundle.

Evenly wrap the roasted vegetable bundles with steak slices. Secure the steak with a toothpick, drizzle with the balsamic glaze and serve.

PER SERVING: Calories: 415, Fat: 22g, Protein: 35g, Sodium: 594mg, Fiber: 2.7g, Carbohydrates: 12g, Sugar: 9.2g

SPAGHETTI SQUASH CAKES

Turn spaghetti squash into crisp and tasty fritters with this simple recipe.

INGREDIENTS

DIRECTIONS

1 spaghetti squash

¼ cup olive oil, divided

1 onion, diced

3 eggs

½ teaspoon sea salt, plus more for seasoning

½ teaspoon freshly ground black pepper, plus more for seasoning

1 tablespoon fresh parsley

Preheat oven to 350 degrees F.

Wash and dry squash thoroughly, then slice in half lengthwise. Scoop out seeds and place both halves on a parchment-lined cookie sheet. Brush the flesh of the squash with oil and season with salt and pepper. Bake cut-side up for about 1 hour, or until squash is fork-tender.

Heat a small skillet coated with oil over medium. Fry the onions for a couple of minutes or until just translucent. Remove from heat.

In a small bowl, mix the eggs together.

Once squash is cool enough to handle, use a fork to separate the squash into "spaghetti" strands and scrape into a bowl. Add the cooked onions, parsley, salt, pepper and eggs. Mix to combine. Form small cakes from the squash mixture.

Heat a large frying pan over medium-low. Coat with olive oil and fry the cakes until browned and crispy on both sides. Drain the cakes on paper towels. Serve with your favorite dipping sauce or Garden Vegetable Spread (page 55).

(Makes about 25 to 30 mini cakes)

PER SERVING: Calories: 168, Fat: 12g, Protein: 4.3g, Sodium: 206mg, Fiber: 2.4g, Carbohydrates: 12g, Sugar: 5g

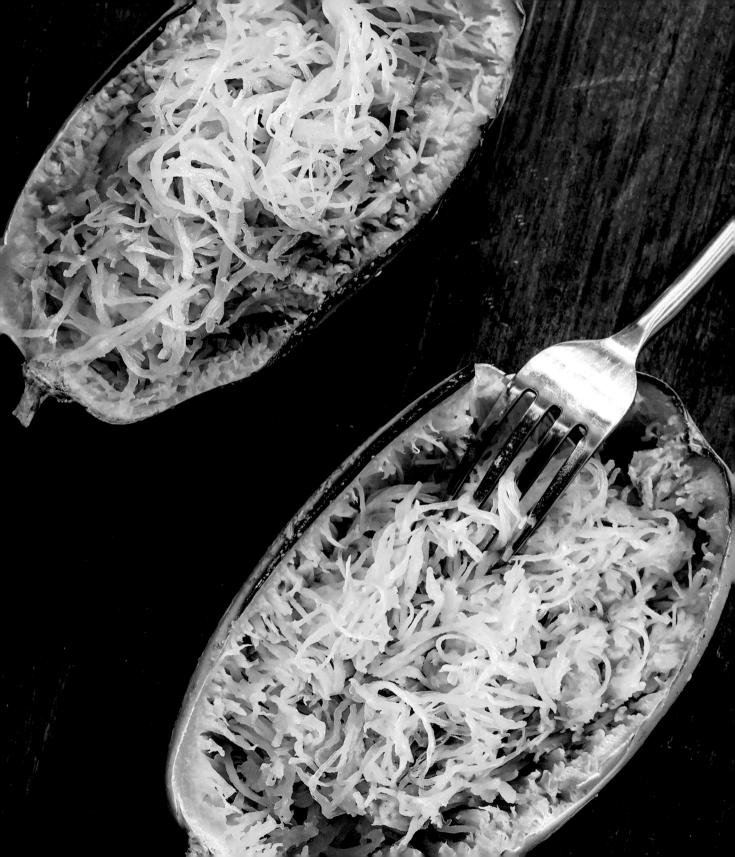

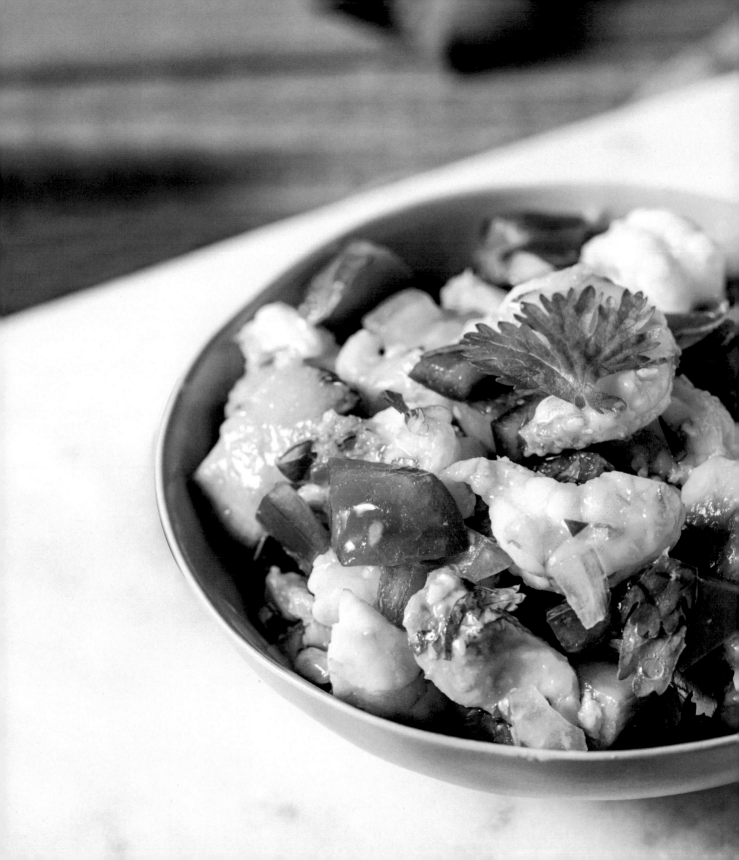

VEGETABLE AND SHRIMP CEVICHE

Healthy and refreshing, ceviche is naturally pegan-friendly—and naturally delightful.

INGREDIENTS

DIRECTIONS

- 1 pound small wild shrimp, diced
- 12 limes, juiced
- 1 tablespoon sea salt
- ½ cup red onion, minced
- 1 ripe avocado, diced
- 1 ripe tomato, seeded and diced
- ½ cup orange pepper, diced
- 1 jalapeño, minced, ½ of seeds removed
- ¼ cup fresh cilantro, finely chopped
- Drizzle olive oil

In a medium shallow glass or ceramic bowl, add the shrimp, lime juice of 10 limes and salt. Mix together, making sure the shrimp is covered with lime juice, adding more if necessary. Place in the refrigerator, covered, for 3 to 4 hours. The lime and salt will "cook" the shrimp.

Take the shrimp from the lime juice mixture and place it in a clean bowl. Add in the remaining lime juice and remaining ingredients and stir to combine. Place the bowl back in the refrigerator for another hour to let the vegetables soften and flavors meld. Place in serving glasses and serve.

PER SERVING: Calories: 196, Fat: 10g, Protein: 17g, Sodium: 1,055mg, Fiber: 2.9g, Carbohydrates: 13g, Sugar: 2.8g

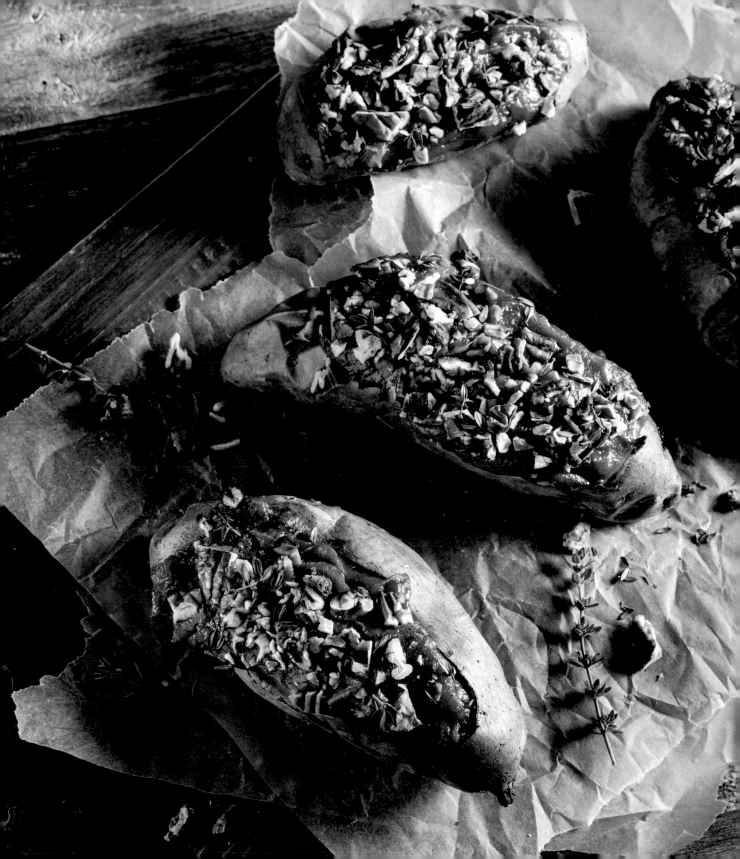

STUFFED SWEET POTATO SNACKS

The combination of sweet potatoes, apples, almond butter and pecans is sweet,
salty and crunchy—so no matter what you're craving, these will hit the spot!

INGREDIENTS	DIRECTIONS	SERVES 4

INGREDIENTS

- 2 small sweet potatoes
- 2 tablespoons almond butter
- 1 honeycrisp apple, cored and diced
- ½ cup pecans, chopped
- ½ tablespoon cinnamon

DIRECTIONS

Preheat oven to 350 degrees F.

Wash the sweet potatoes and prick with a fork. Wrap each potato in foil and cook until tender, about 40 to 45 minutes.

Cut the cooked potatoes in half lengthwise. Make a slice in the middle of each potato and open slightly by squeezing the ends together. Place ½ tablespoon almond butter in each potato, top with diced apples, an even amount of pecans and sprinkle with cinnamon.

PER SERVING: Calories: 220, Fat: 14g, Protein: 4.1g, Sodium: 36mg, Fiber: 5.7g, Carbohydrates: 23g, Sugar: 7.8g

STEAMED CHICKEN AND VEGETABLE PINWHEELS

These pinwheels are a fun appetizer that presents beautifully. Make it your own by switching up the Italian seasoning with Middle Eastern za'atar or Spanish smoked paprika.

INGREDIENTS

1 tablespoon olive oil

1 onion, diced

3 cups spinach

1½ pounds chicken, cooked and diced

1 cup roasted red peppers, diced

2 tablespoons fresh parsley, chopped

1½ tablespoons Italian seasoning

1 teaspoon salt

1 teaspoon pepper

2 large yellow squash

4 large carrots

Small bundle fresh chives

2 cups marinara sauce

DIRECTIONS

Heat a sauté pan over medium-low. Add oil and sauté the onions until softened. Add spinach and cook until wilted.

In a medium bowl, mix together the chicken, onions, spinach, red peppers, parsley, Italian seasoning, salt and pepper.

Using a mandolin, carefully slice the squash and carrots lengthwise in strips.

With a vegetable steamer, steam the squash and carrots until just soft and pliable.

Take a squash strip, top it with a carrot strip, place the chicken and spinach mixture on top, roll up and tie with chives to keep closed.

Steam the bundles until vegetables are soft and filling is hot, about 5 minutes.

Heat up the sauce and place on a serving platter. Place the bundles on top and serve.

SERVES 6-8

PER SERVING: Calories: 255, Fat: 5.6g, Protein: 29g, Sodium: 883mg, Fiber: 4.2g, Carbohydrates: 19g, Sugar: 10g

VEGETABLE-STUFFED ARTICHOKES

Preparing your own artichokes can be a little time-consuming, but the beautiful presentation and amazing taste is more than worth it.

INGREDIENTS

- 4 artichokes
- 1 lemon
- ½ cup kale
- ½ yellow pepper
- ½ cup purple cabbage
- 1 carrot
- 2 garlic cloves
- 4 sardine fillets
- ½ tablespoon olive oil
- ¼ teaspoon sea salt
- ¼ teaspoon freshly ground black pepper

DIRECTIONS

Preheat oven to 425 degrees F.

Wash the artichokes thoroughly. Cut the stems off the bottoms of the artichoke. With scissors, snip off the tip of each artichoke petal, then cut the top of the artichoke off. Cut the lemon in half and rub lemon on the cut areas of the artichoke to prevent browning.

Finely mince all vegetables and sardines. In a medium bowl, stir the minced mixture together with olive oil, salt and pepper. Open artichokes and fill each petal with the vegetable mixture.

Wrap each stuffed artichoke with foil and place in the preheated oven. Bake for 1 hour and 20 minutes, or until leaves release easily when pulled.

SERVES 4

PER SERVING: Calories: 155, Fat: 5g, Protein: 12g, Sodium: 333mg, Fiber: 8.2g, Carbohydrates: 19g, Sugar: 3g

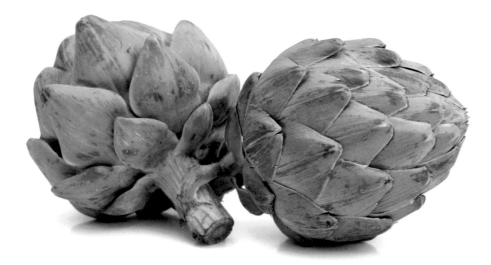

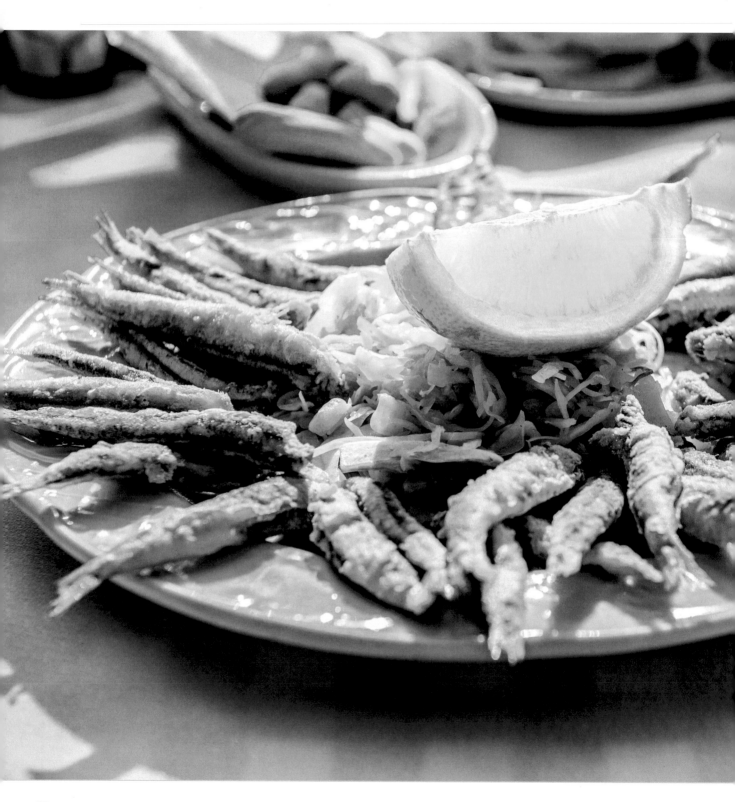

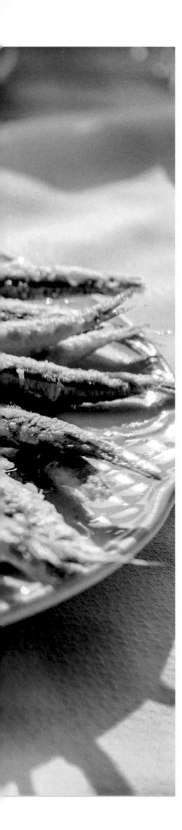

FRIED ANCHOVIES

Don't let anchovies scare you—when cooked, they have a wonderfully nutty flavor. Frying anchovies is a great way to introduce this superfood packed with omega-3 fatty acids. You can eat them plain, top your salad with them or serve them as an appetizer with a dip.

INGREDIENTS	DIRECTIONS	SERVES 4

INGREDIENTS

- 1½ pounds prepared anchovies, canned
- 2 eggs
- 1 cup coconut flour
- 1 teaspoon freshly ground black pepper
- ½ teaspoon red pepper flakes
- Zest of 1 lemon
- Olive oil, for frying

DIRECTIONS

Pat the anchovies dry with a paper towel.

In a medium shallow bowl, mix the eggs together.

In another medium shallow bowl, mix together the flour, pepper, red pepper and zest.

Dip the anchovies in the eggs and then in the flour mixture. Set aside.

Heat ½-inch oil in a large skillet until shimmering. Fry the anchovies until golden brown, about 2 minutes on each side. Drain on paper towels.

PER SERVING: Calories: 412, Fat: 18g, Protein: 42g, Sodium: 272mg, Fiber: 10g, Carbohydrates: 17g, Sugar: 2.5g

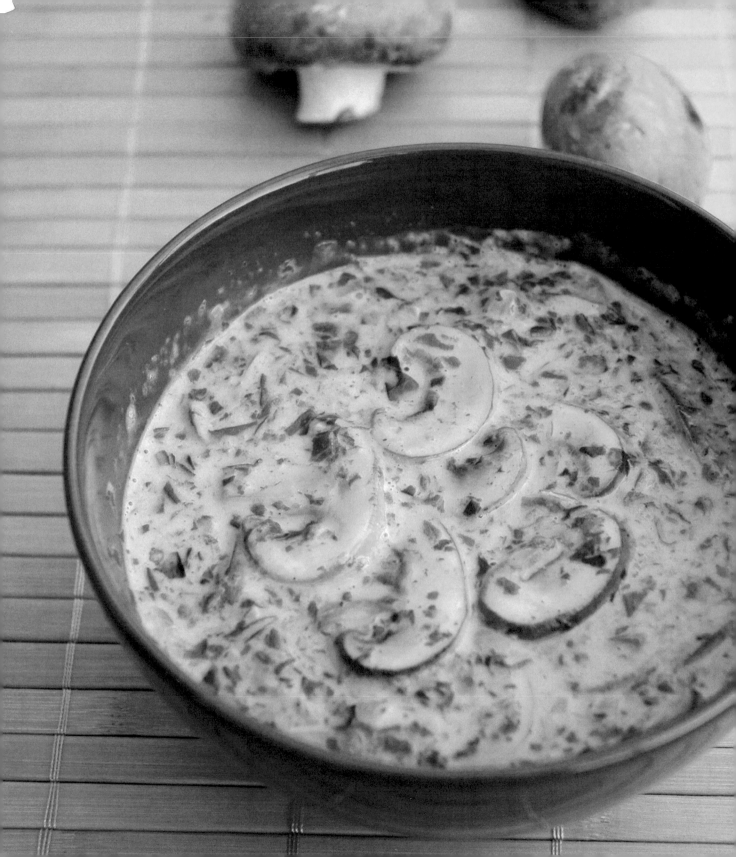

soups & salads

LOAD UP ON LIGHTER FARE.

Buffalo Chicken Soup 97

Easy Vegetable Bean Soup 97

Summer Salad 98

Brussels Sprout and Beet Salad with
Lemon Poppy Seed Dressing 99

Arugula Cucumber Gazpacho 101

Brussels Sprout Salad 102

Frisée, Grapefruit and Long Bean Salad with
Warm Anchovy, Orange and Herb Dressing 104

Kale, Blood Orange and Pomegranate Salad
with Ginger Carrot Dressing 105

Butternut Squash Soup with Cajun Prawns 107

Romaine Wedge Salad with Lemon, Basil
and Flaxseed Dressing 108

Cucumber Spiral Salad 109

Lemon Ginger Avgolemono 110

Grilled Radicchio and Pear Salad with
Warm Bacon Dressing 112

Carrot Ginger Soup 115

Arugula, Raspberry and Hazelnut Salad 115

Tri-Beet Salad 117

Hearty Mushroom and Spinach Soup 118

Vegetable Quinoa Salad 121

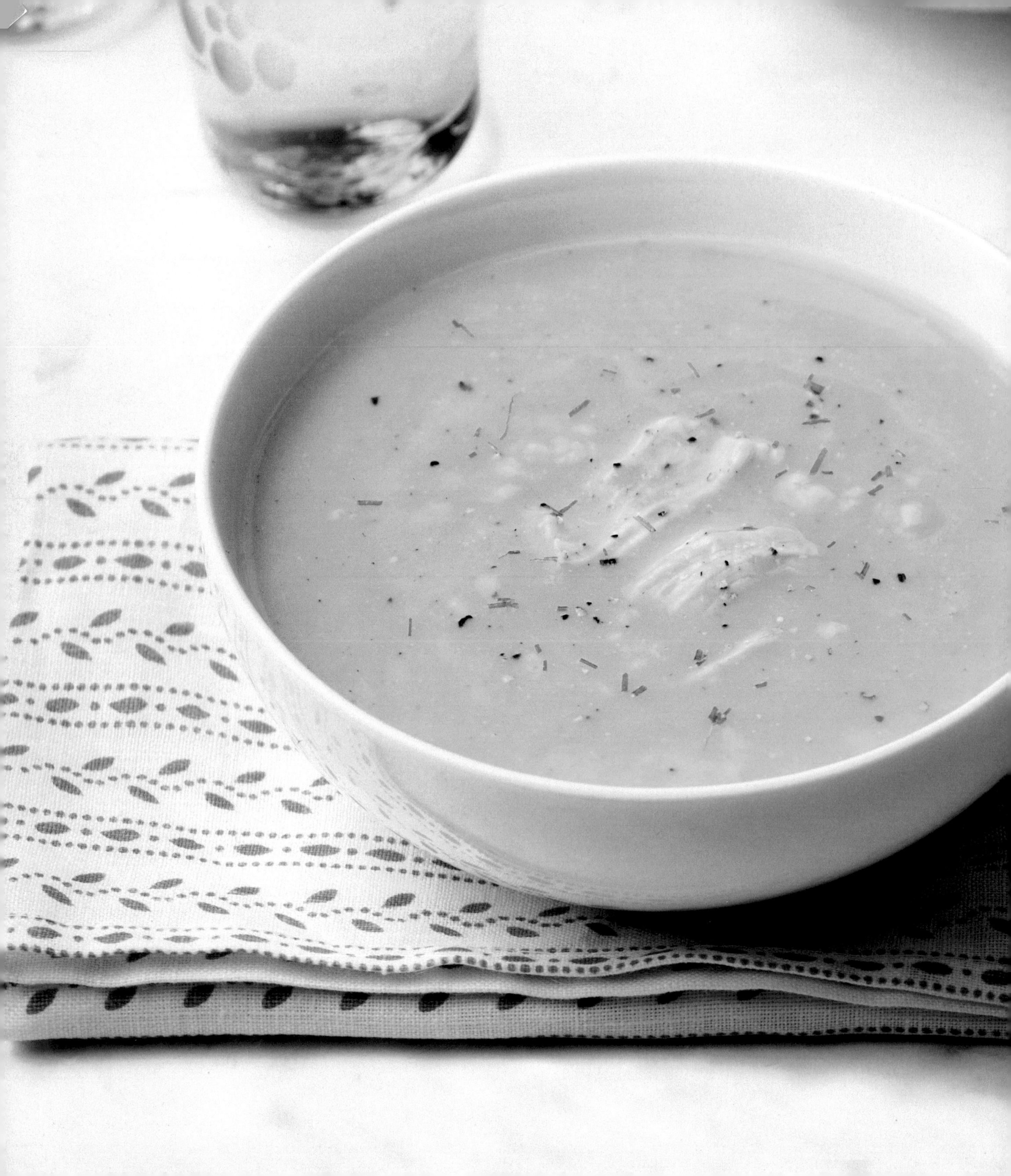

BUFFALO CHICKEN SOUP

This beautiful bowl of soup evokes the flavors of everyone's favorite game-day snack without weighing you down with oil and blue cheese.

INGREDIENTS	DIRECTIONS	SERVES 4

INGREDIENTS

2 tablespoons olive oil

1 stalk celery, diced, plus extra for garnish

1 small onion, diced

1 carrot, diced, plus extra for garnish

5 cups vegetable broth

¼ cup hot sauce

1 cup sheep's yogurt

3 cups cooked chicken, chopped

DIRECTIONS

In a soup pot over medium heat, add the oil and cook the celery, onions and carrots until just softened, about 5 minutes.

Add in the broth. Simmer for 10 to 15 minutes to reduce the liquid and meld flavors. Use an immersion blender to blend the broth until smooth and add the hot sauce. Place the yogurt in a medium bowl. Slowly add 2 cups broth to the yogurt and whisk the two together—this will keep the yogurt from curdling. Slowly stir the yogurt mixture into the rest of the broth.

Divide the soup between four serving bowls. Place an even amount of chicken into the middle of each and top with the diced celery and carrots if desired.

PER SERVING: Calories: 314, Fat: 12g, Protein: 43g, Sodium: 899mg, Fiber: 2.2g, Carbohydrates: 11g, Sugar: 5.2g

EASY VEGETABLE BEAN SOUP

If you have leftover Vegetable Chop (page 146), this soup can be ready in 15 minutes.

INGREDIENTS	DIRECTIONS	SERVES 4

INGREDIENTS

3 cups Vegetable Chop (page 146)

1 can red beans, drained

6 cups vegetable broth

DIRECTIONS

Simmer all ingredients in a soup pot over medium heat until hot and the broth has reduced a little to enhance the flavor, about 10 minutes.

PER SERVING: Calories: 205, Fat: 5.4g, Protein: 11g, Sodium: 456mg, Fiber: 11g, Carbohydrates: 31g, Sugar: 5.9g

SUMMER SALAD

This light, bright and refreshing salad could not be simpler to put together.

INGREDIENTS

DIRECTIONS

- 2 cups grape tomatoes, cut in half
- 1 English cucumber, peeled, seeded, diced
- 1 avocado, diced
- 2 tablespoons diced red onion
- ¼ cup fresh basil
- 1 tablespoon fresh parsley, minced
- ½ teaspoon sea salt
- ½ teaspoon freshly ground black pepper
- 3 tablespoons olive oil
- 1 tablespoon red wine vinegar
- 3 ounces goat cheese, crumbled

In a large bowl, add all ingredients except the goat cheese and gently stir to combine. Divide the salad among four plates and top with the crumbled goat cheese.

PER SERVING: Calories: 284, Fat: 24g, Protein: 8.8g, Sodium: 320mg, Fiber: 4.3g, Carbohydrates: 9.6g, Sugar: 2.7g

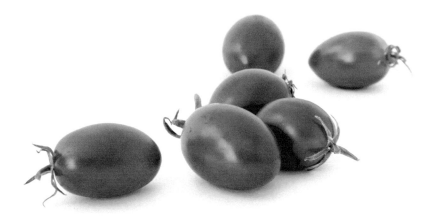

BRUSSELS SPROUT AND BEET SALAD WITH LEMON POPPY SEED DRESSING

This salad's bright citrus dressing livens up the earthiness from the beets and Brussels sprouts.

| INGREDIENTS | DIRECTIONS | SERVES 4 |

INGREDIENTS

SALAD

- 1 small yellow beet
- 1 tablespoon olive oil
- 2 cups kale, thinly sliced
- ½ cup red cabbage, thinly sliced
- ½ cup Napa cabbage, thinly sliced
- 2 cups butter lettuce, chopped
- 2 cups Brussels sprouts, roasted

LEMON POPPY SEED DRESSING

- ½ lemon, juice and zest
- 2 tablespoons white balsamic vinegar
- ½ teaspoon sea salt
- ½ teaspoon freshly ground pepper
- ½ cup olive oil
- 1½ teaspoons poppy seeds

DIRECTIONS

Preheat oven to 350 degrees F.

Peel the beet, drizzle with oil and wrap in foil. Bake for 40 minutes, or until fork-tender. Take the beet out and let cool.

Wash and dry all of the lettuce and cabbage. Slice the beet in thin rounds.

In a medium jar with a lid, add all dressing ingredients and shake to mix.

Arrange the salad on a serving dish. Top the salad with beets and Brussels sprouts. Drizzle the desired amount of dressing onto the salad and serve.

PER SERVING: SALAD: Calories: 83, Fat: 3.9g, Protein: 3.9g, Sodium: 45mg, Fiber: 4.2g, Carbohydrates: 11g, Sugar: 4g **DRESSING:** Calories: 254, Fat: 27.5g, Protein: 0.3g, Sodium: 223mg, Fiber: 0.3g, Carbohydrates: 2.3g, Sugar: 1.4g

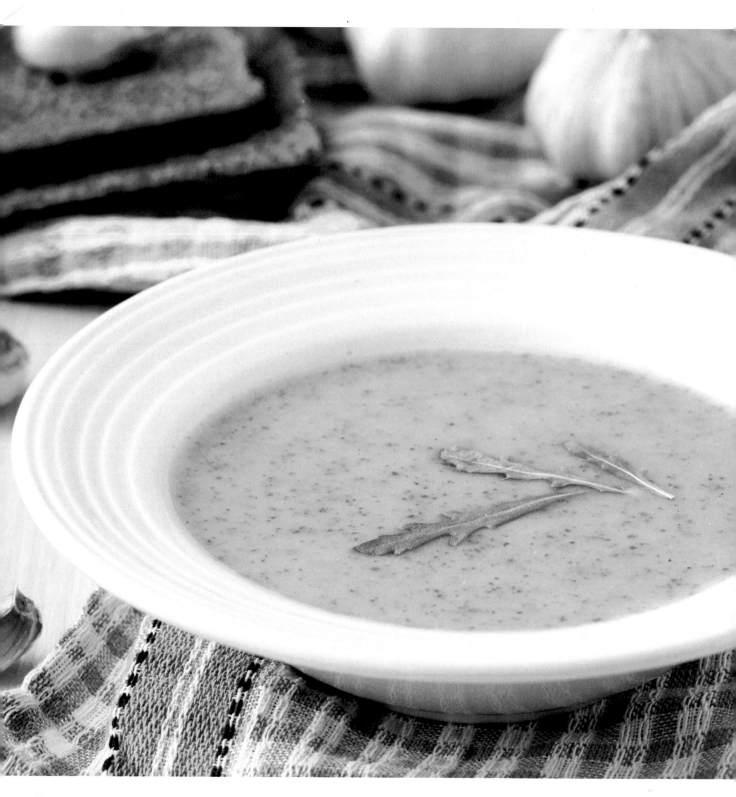

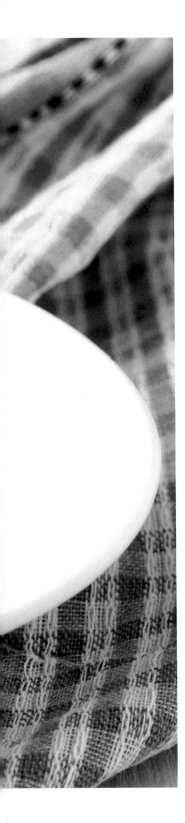

ARUGULA CUCUMBER GAZPACHO

This scrumptious soup gives you a peppery bite from the arugula and a little heat from the jalapeño, balanced by the cool refreshing taste of cucumber.

INGREDIENTS	DIRECTIONS	SERVES 4

INGREDIENTS

- 1 English cucumber, chopped
- 1 lime, juiced
- 2 cups arugula, washed, plus extra for garnish
- 2 tablespoons apple cider vinegar
- 1 clove garlic, minced
- ¼ cup green onions, chopped
- ½ teaspoon sea salt
- 1 jalapeño, seeded
- Water

DIRECTIONS

Blend all soup ingredients in a blender, adding water as you blend until you reach a smooth soup with the consistency of heavy cream. Evenly pour it into four bowls, garnish with arugula and serve.

PER SERVING: Calories: 16, Fat: 0.2g, Protein: 0.7g, Sodium: 225mg, Fiber: 0.7g, Carbohydrates: 3.8g, Sugar: 1.7g

BRUSSELS SPROUT SALAD

Featuring shaved Brussels sprouts and an apple-mustard dressing, this salad is just right for fall.

| INGREDIENTS | DIRECTIONS | SERVES 4 |

SALAD

1½ pounds Brussels sprouts

½ cup pomegranate seeds

½ cup pistachios

DRESSING

½ sweet apple, peeled and chopped

½ shallot, minced

1½ teaspoons Dijon mustard

6 tablespoons olive oil

1½ tablespoons apple cider vinegar

1½ teaspoons lemon juice

Cut the ends off of each sprout and slice thinly lengthwise to make shreds. Wash and dry the sprouts.

Place all salad dressing ingredients in a blender and blend until smooth.

Arrange the Brussels sprouts, pomegranate seeds and pistachios on a serving plate. Drizzle the salad dressing over the salad and serve.

PER SERVING: SALAD: Calories: 129, Fat: 4.2g, Protein: 7.5g, Sodium: 43mg, Fiber: 8g, Carbohydrates: 20g, Sugar: 6.6g
DRESSING: Calories: 194, Fat: 20.5g, Protein: 0.2g, Sodium: 31mg, Fiber: 0.6g, Carbohydrates: 3.4g, Sugar: 2.3g

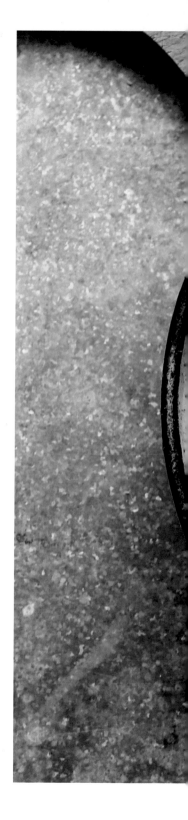

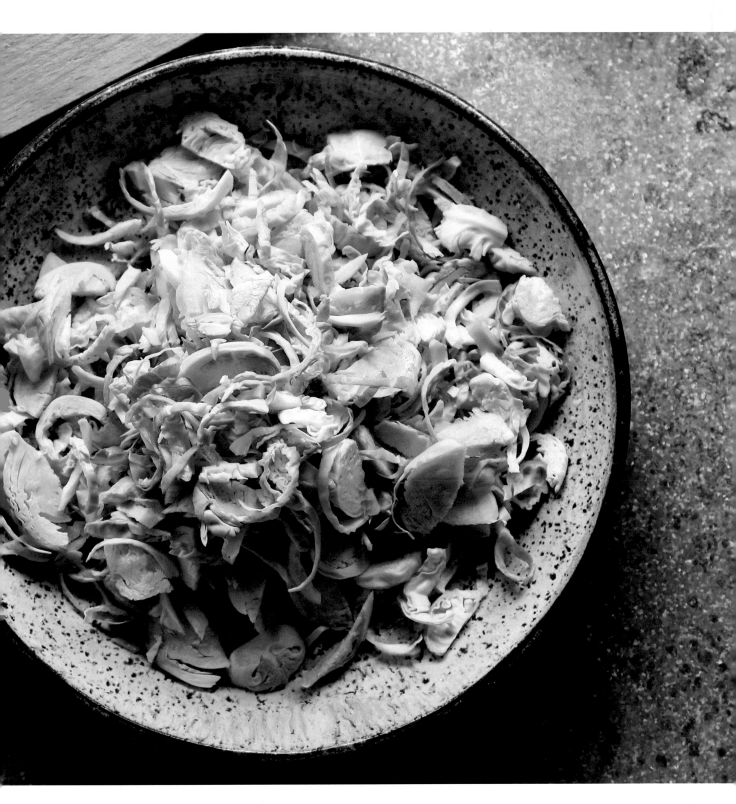

FRISÉE, GRAPEFRUIT AND LONG BEAN SALAD WITH WARM ANCHOVY, ORANGE AND HERB DRESSING

This fun salad is a perfect example of how healthy eating doesn't have to be boring—and can definitely be delicious.

INGREDIENTS | **DIRECTIONS** | **SERVES 4**

SALAD

- 1 head frisée lettuce
- 1 grapefruit
- ½ cup walnuts
- ½ pound Chinese long beans, trimmed
- 2 tablespoons olive oil
- ½ teaspoon sea salt
- ¼ teaspoon freshly ground black pepper

WARM ANCHOVY, ORANGE AND HERB DRESSING

- 6 tablespoons olive oil, divided
- ¼ shallot, minced
- 1 clove garlic, minced
- 2 anchovy fillets
- ¼ teaspoon freshly ground black pepper
- 1½ teaspoons fresh parsley, chopped
- ½ tablespoon fresh oregano, chopped
- 1¼ teaspoons fresh basil, chopped
- ¼ teaspoon fresh thyme, chopped
- 2 tablespoons white wine vinegar
- ½ orange, juice and zest

Wash and trim the lettuce and set aside.

To segment the grapefruit, on a cutting board, cut off the ends of the grapefruit. Place a cut-end down onto the cutting board and slice off the grapefruit peel by slicing down from the top around the grapefruit. Cut into the grapefruit next to the pith to remove segments.

In a small frying pan over medium-low heat, toast the walnuts for about 3 minutes, or until just toasted, and set aside. Remove from the pan.

In a large frying pan over medium heat, add the oil and cook the beans for about 6 minutes, stirring often. Season with salt and pepper.

In the same small frying pan over medium heat, add 1 tablespoon oil. Cook the shallot, garlic and anchovies for about 3 minutes, or until the anchovies have melted, mashing the anchovies up with a wooden spoon while cooking. Add the herbs in the last minute of cooking.

In a glass container or jar with a lid, add the remaining oil, vinegar and the orange juice. Add the anchovy mix to the container and shake to combine.

Transfer the cooked beans to a large serving platter. Arrange the lettuce on the platter, top with the grapefruit sections and toasted walnuts. Drizzle the dressing on and garnish with the orange zest.

PER SERVING: SALAD: Calories: 225, Fat: 17g, Protein: 6.1g, Sodium: 220mg, Fiber: 1.7g, Carbohydrates: 16g, Sugar: 0.4g **DRESSING:** Calories: 189, Fat: 20.5g, Protein: 0.4g, Sodium: 59mg, Fiber: 0.2g, Carbohydrates: 1.8g, Sugar: 1.1g

KALE, BLOOD ORANGE AND POMEGRANATE SALAD WITH GINGER CARROT DRESSING

This colorful salad is as tasty as it is healthy! It also makes a great lunch to pack for work—kale is one of the few salad greens that won't get soggy after a few hours.

INGREDIENTS   **DIRECTIONS**   SERVES 4

SALAD

- 1 large bunch kale
- 1 blood orange
- ½ red onion, sliced thin
- ½ cup pomegranate seeds

DRESSING

- ¼ cup olive oil
- 2 tablespoons white balsamic vinegar
- ½ teaspoon pure honey
- ½ tablespoon finely grated ginger
- ⅛ teaspoon freshly ground black pepper
- ¼ cup grated carrot

Wash and dry the kale and remove the stems. Chop the kale into a large chiffonade by placing the kale leaves on top of each other, rolling them together and cutting the roll into ½-inch slices.

On a cutting board, cut off the ends of the orange. Place a cut-end down and slice off the orange peel by slicing down from the top around the orange. Cut into the orange next to the pith sections to remove the orange sections.

Place the kale on a serving dish. Top with the segmented orange, onions and pomegranate seeds.

Mix all salad dressing ingredients in a blender. Dress the salad with the dressing and serve.

PER SERVING: SALAD: Calories: 62, Fat: 0.6g, Protein: 2.8g, Sodium: 19mg, Fiber: 3.5g, Carbohydrates: 13g, Sugar: 6.9g **DRESSING:** Calories: 133, Fat: 13.5g, Protein: 0.2g, Sodium: 7.5mg, Fiber: 0.3g, Carbohydrates: 2.8g, Sugar: 2.3g

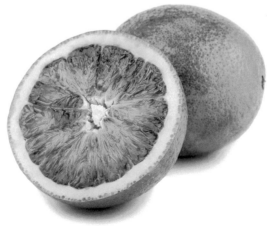

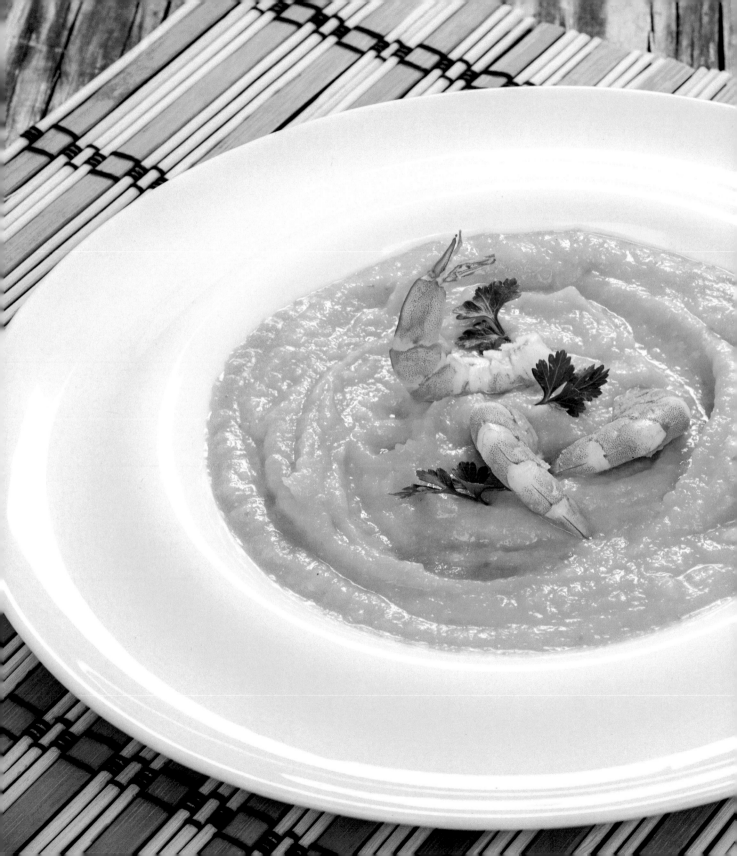

BUTTERNUT SQUASH SOUP WITH CAJUN PRAWNS

This soup is just right for a cold winter's night—the hot soup and slight heat from the Cajun prawns will warm you up!

INGREDIENTS

DIRECTIONS

SOUP

- 1 butternut squash
- 1 honeycrisp apple
- 2 tablespoons olive oil
- 1 onion, diced
- 2 stalks celery, diced
- 3 cloves garlic, minced
- 2 carrots, diced
- 6 cups vegetable broth
- ¼ teaspoon fresh sage, minced
- ¼ teaspoon freshly grated nutmeg
- ¼ teaspoon pumpkin spice
- ¼ teaspoon sea salt
- ¼ teaspoon freshly ground black pepper
- 1 cup unsweetened coconut milk

CAJUN PRAWNS

- 12 jumbo prawns, peeled with tails on
- 1 tablespoon olive oil
- 1 tablespoon Cajun seasoning

GARNISH

- 8 fresh sage leaves
- 1 tablespoon olive oil
- ¼ cup sheep's yogurt

Preheat oven to 325 degrees F.

Wash and peel the squash and apple. Cut the squash in half lengthwise and scoop out the seeds. Cut the squash into 1-inch pieces. Cut the apple in half and remove the core. Place the squash and apple on a parchment-lined cookie sheet, drizzle with 1 tablespoon olive oil and season with salt and pepper. Roast in the preheated oven for about 20 minutes, or until the apple and squash are fork-tender.

Meanwhile, in a large pot over medium heat with 1 tablespoon olive oil, cook the onions, garlic, carrots and celery until vegetables are soft, about 5 minutes. Add in the broth and season with the sage, nutmeg, pumpkin spice, salt and pepper. Add the cooked apple and squash to the soup. Simmer the soup for 20 minutes. Add the coconut milk and heat through.

Purée soup with an immersion blender until smooth.

In a medium bowl, mix together the shrimp and Cajun seasoning. In a nonstick skillet with 1 tablespoon olive oil, cook the prawns until pink and no longer opaque, about 3 minutes on each side.

Add the remaining olive oil to a small saucepan over medium heat. Cook the sage leaves until just crisp. Drain on paper towels.

Place the soup in four serving bowls and set three prawns on top of each bowl of soup. Garnish with the yogurt and fried sage leaves.

PER SERVING: Calories: 462, Fat: 24g, Protein: 8.4g, Sodium: 430mg, Fiber: 11g, Carbohydrates: 60g, Sugar: 19g

ROMAINE WEDGE SALAD WITH LEMON, BASIL AND FLAXSEED DRESSING

Classic wedge salads drenched in blue cheese and bacon are overrated—try this light and flavorful wedge salad instead.

INGREDIENTS

DIRECTIONS

SERVES 4

SALAD

- 2 small heads romaine lettuce
- 2 cups ripe plums, diced
- 1 red chili pepper, seeded, minced
- 1 cup cherry tomatoes, halved
- ½ cup English cucumber, chopped

LEMON, BASIL, FLAXSEED DRESSING

- 1 tablespoon finely ground flaxseed
- ¼ cup water
- Juice of ¼ lemon
- 1½ teaspoons fresh basil, chopped
- ½ teaspoon white balsamic vinegar
- ¼ teaspoon sea salt
- ⅛ teaspoon freshly ground black pepper

Trim the lettuce heads, removing the outer leaves and end of the stem, making sure the core is still intact. Cut the lettuce heads in half lengthwise. Wash the lettuce thoroughly and dry. Set aside.

In a small bowl, mix together the plums, pepper, tomatoes and cucumber. Set aside.

In a container or jar with a lid, add the flaxseed and water and let set for 5 minutes. Add the remaining salad dressing ingredients and shake to combine.

Place each lettuce wedge on a plate. Top each evenly with the plum mixture, drizzle with the desired amount of dressing and serve.

PER SERVING: SALAD: Calories: 80, Fat: 0.7g, Protein: 3g, Sodium: 17mg, Fiber: 4.4g, Carbohydrates: 18g, Sugar: 12g **DRESSING:** Calories: 10, Fat: 0.6g, Protein: 0.4g, Sodium: 110.5mg, Fiber: 0.4g, Carbohydrates: 0.8g, Sugar: 0.2g

CUCUMBER SPIRAL SALAD

This light, bright and summery salad is impossibly easy to throw together, making it perfect for any occasion—especially a last-minute one.

| INGREDIENTS | DIRECTIONS | SERVES 4 |

SALAD

- 3 sweet apples
- 1½ English cucumber
- ½ red onion, thinly sliced
- Juice of ½ lemon

DRESSING

- 6 tablespoons sheep's yogurt
- Zest of ½ lemon
- 1 tablespoon fresh dill, chopped, extra for garnish
- 1½ teaspoons apple cider vinegar
- ¼ teaspoon sea salt
- ¼ teaspoon freshly ground black pepper

To core the apples, place them on a cutting board, place the apple corer on top of each stem and push down through the apple before pulling up to remove the core. Use a paring knife to remove any remaining seeds or core, if any.

Using a spiralizer, slice the cucumbers and apples. If you don't have a spiralizer, you can thinly slice the cucumbers and apples by hand or with a mandolin slicer.

Place the sliced apples in a large bowl, add the onions and lemon juice and gently toss to coat. Add the sliced cucumber to the bowl.

In a small bowl, mix together the yogurt, lemon zest, dill, vinegar, salt and pepper. Pour the mixture over the cucumbers and apples, toss to coat and serve.

PER SERVING: SALAD: Calories: 68, Fat: 0.3g, Protein: 0.9g, Sodium: 2.5mg, Fiber: 3g, Carbohydrates: 18g, Sugar: 12g **DRESSING:** Calories: 19.5, Fat: 1.3g, Protein: 1.3g, Sodium: 118mg, Fiber: 0g, Carbohydrates: 1.4g, Sugar: 0.6g

LEMON GINGER AVGOLEMONO

Avgolemono is a traditional Greek soup consisting of egg yolk and lemon. This version adds ginger and a few other ingredients for a tasty twist on the classic.

| INGREDIENTS | DIRECTIONS | SERVES 4 |

INGREDIENTS

- 1 tablespoon olive oil
- 1 onion, diced
- 2 cloves garlic, minced
- 6 cups chicken broth or vegetable broth
- 3 eggs
- 3 cups cooked chicken
- 1 tablespoon grated fresh ginger
- 1 teaspoon sea salt
- 1 teaspoon freshly ground black pepper
- 3 cups Cauliflower Rice (page 129)
- 2 lemons, juice and zest
- 4 sprigs of fresh parsley, chopped

DIRECTIONS

In a large soup pot over medium heat, add the oil and cook the onions and garlic until tender, about 3 to 4 minutes. Add in the broth and bring to a simmer.

In a medium bowl, whisk the eggs.

Slowly pour 1 cup hot broth into the eggs while whisking vigorously. Slowly whisk the egg mixture back into the soup. Add the chicken, ginger, salt, pepper and cauliflower rice. Continue to cook another couple of minutes. Remove from heat and add the lemon juice and lemon zest. Garnish with parsley and serve.

PER SERVING: Calories: 326, Fat: 9.5g, Protein: 47g, Sodium: 806mg, Fiber: 2.8g, Carbohydrates: 13g, Sugar: 5.6g

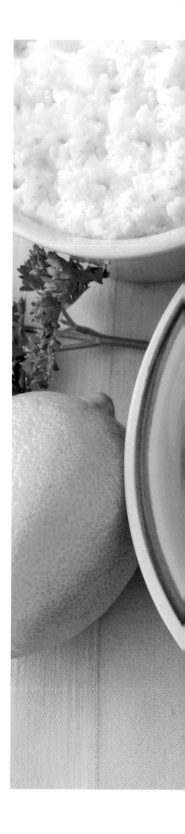

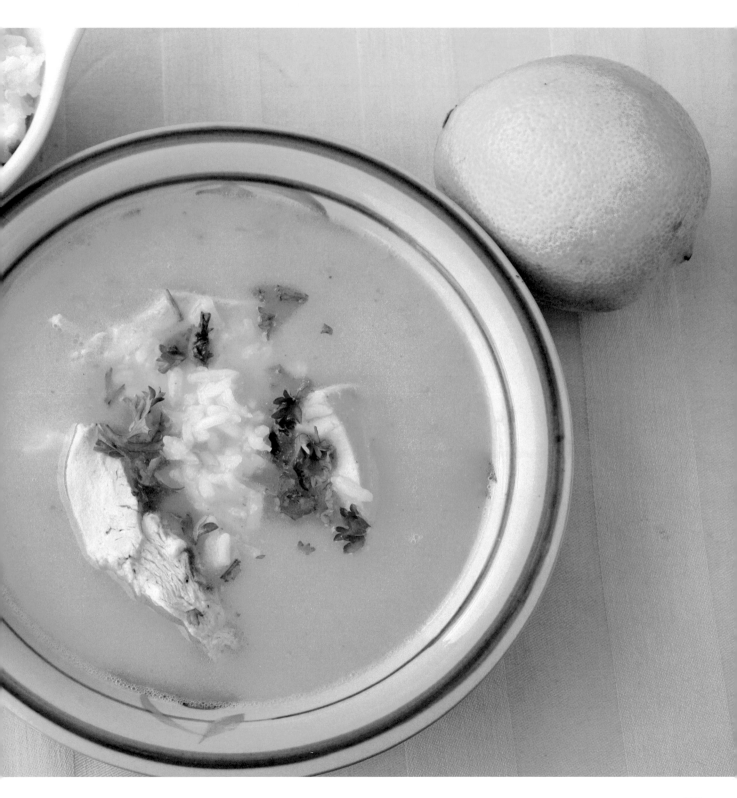

GRILLED RADICCHIO AND PEAR SALAD WITH WARM BACON DRESSING

Radicchio is a member of the chicory family, meaning it's packed with antioxidants and high in fiber but can be bitter if not cooked or grilled. Serve this salad alongside grilled meats for a hearty dinner.

| INGREDIENTS | DIRECTIONS | SERVES 4 |

SALAD

- 2 heads radicchio
- 3 ripe pears
- 1 tablespoon olive oil

DRESSING

- 2½ slices bacon
- ½ shallot, minced
- 1 tablespoon apple cider vinegar
- 1½ teaspoons whole grain mustard

Preheat grill to medium heat.

Cut the radicchio in half lengthwise. Wash and dry the radicchio and trim the core, leaving the core attached.

Cut the pears in half and scoop out the core. Brush radicchio and pears with oil and place on a hot grill cut-side down. Grill until grill marks appear, the pears are just softened and the radicchio is slightly charred and wilted. Slice the pears into thin slices.

In a nonstick pan over medium heat, cook the bacon until browned and crisp. Drain on paper towels. Reserve 2 tablespoons bacon grease, add the shallot and cook for a couple of minutes. Stir in the vinegar and mustard and mix. Cut the bacon into small pieces and add to the dressing.

Transfer all dressing ingredients into a container with a top. Shake to mix.

Place the radicchio on a serving dish, top with the pear slices, pour the dressing over the salad and serve.

PER SERVING: SALAD: Calories: 122, Fat: 3.8g, Protein: 1.8g, Sodium: 22mg, Fiber: 4.7g, Carbohydrates: 23g, Sugar: 13g **DRESSING:** Calories: 34, Fat: 2.4g, Protein: 1.7g, Sodium: 105.5mg, Fiber: 0.2g, Carbohydrates: 0.9g, Sugar: 0.4g

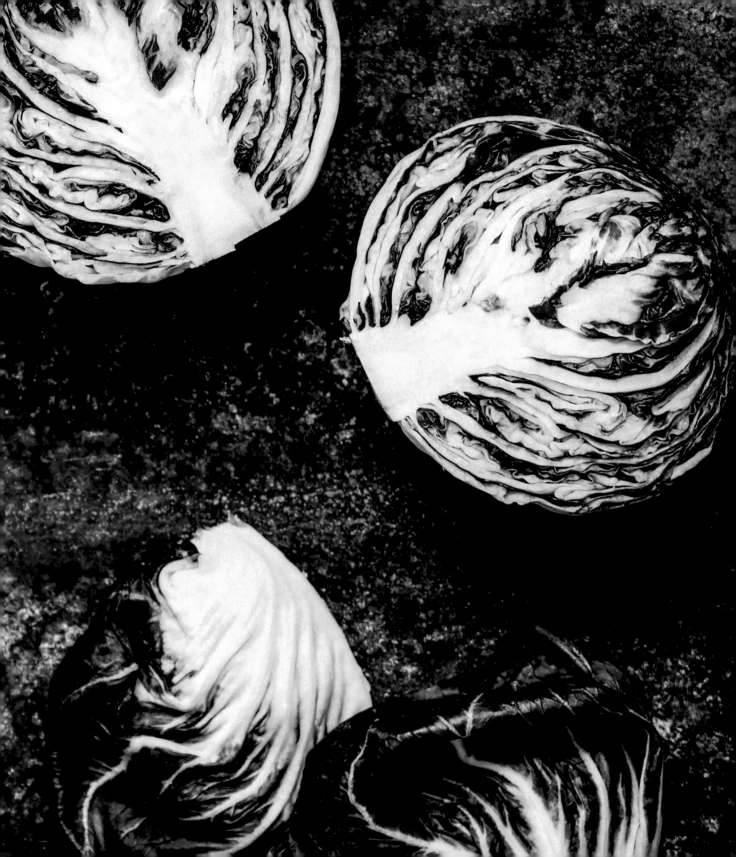

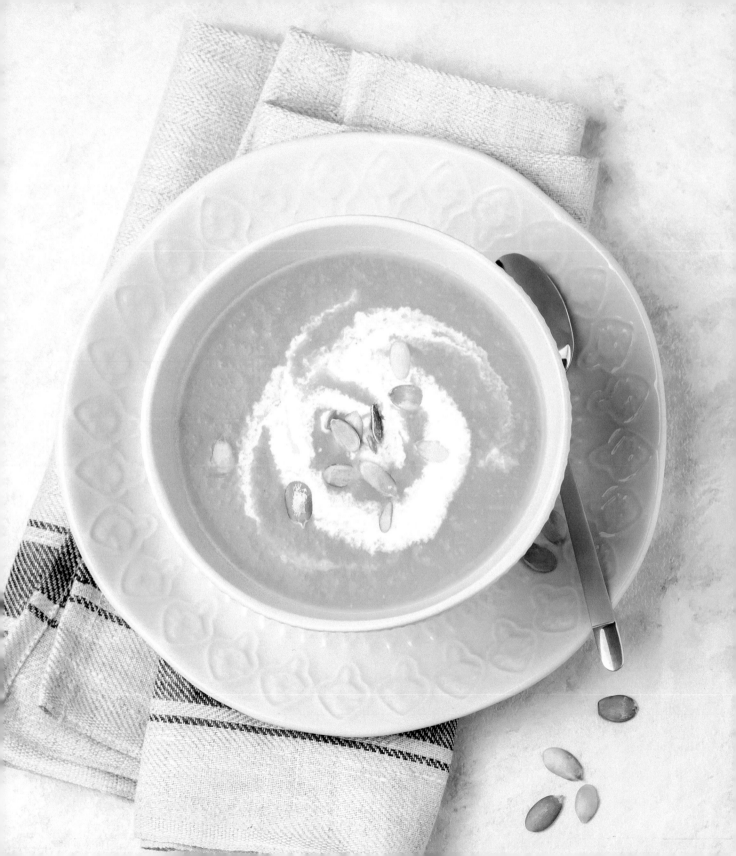

CARROT GINGER SOUP

Sweet, spicy and a little creamy, this simple soup will have you coming back for more. Don't skip the toasted pepitas—they add a wonderful crunch.

INGREDIENTS | DIRECTIONS | SERVES 4

INGREDIENTS

- 4 large carrots
- 1 teaspoon turmeric
- 1 teaspoon five-spice
- 1 tablespoon grated ginger
- Pinch of cayenne pepper
- 6 cups vegetable broth
- ⅓ cup pepitas
- ½ cup sheep's yogurt

DIRECTIONS

Peel and chop the carrots. Add carrots into a large soup pot over medium-low heat and add remaining soup ingredients except the pepitas and yogurt. Simmer the soup until the carrots are fork-tender, about 15 to 20 minutes.

In a small saucepan over medium heat, toast the pepitas slightly.

Blend the soup in a blender or with an immersion blender until smooth. Divide the soup evenly into four serving bowls, garnish with an even amount of yogurt and pepitas in each.

PER SERVING: Calories: 96, Fat: 2.7g, Protein: 4.4g, Sodium: 271mg, Fiber: 3.8g, Carbohydrates: 13g, Sugar: 7g

ARUGULA, RASPBERRY AND HAZELNUT SALAD

This simple combination of raspberries, arugula and hazelnuts makes for a salad that is sweet, savory and crunchy.

INGREDIENTS | DIRECTIONS | SERVES 4

INGREDIENTS

SALAD

- ⅓ cup hazelnuts
- 8 ounces arugula
- 1 pint fresh raspberries

DRESSING

- ¼ cup olive oil
- 2 tablespoons lime juice
- 1 tablespoon cilantro, chopped fine
- ½ small shallot, minced
- 1½ teaspoons apple cider vinegar

DIRECTIONS

Add the hazelnuts to a small nonstick pan over medium-low heat and lightly toast, stirring often, about 2 to 3 minutes.

Wash and dry the arugula. Arrange the arugula on a serving plate. Top with the raspberries and hazelnuts.

Add all salad dressing ingredients together in a jar with a lid and shake until combined. Pour the dressing onto the salad and serve.

PER SERVING: SALAD: Calories: 112, Fat: 7.3g, Protein: 2.7g, Sodium: 2.1mg, Fiber: 6.2g, Carbohydrates: 11g, Sugar: 4g **DRESSING:** Calories: 125, Fat: 13.5g, Protein: 0.2g, Sodium: 1.2mg, Fiber: 0.2g, Carbohydrates: 1.6g, Sugar: 0.6g

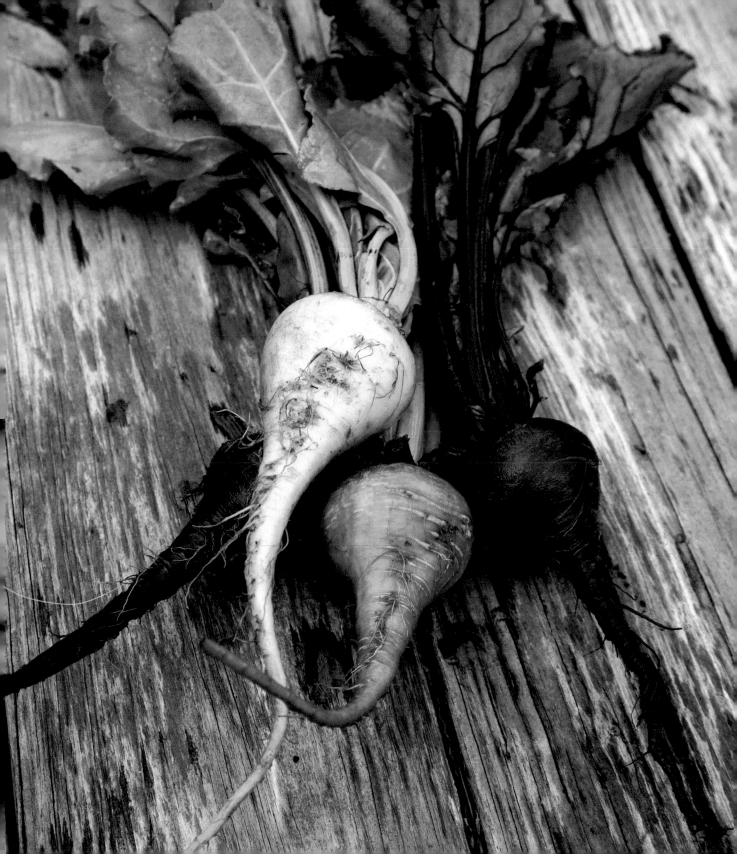

TRI-BEET SALAD

This stunning salad will impress with presentation and flavor! Beets are low in calories and a great source of nutrients, making them a very beneficial addition to your diet.

INGREDIENTS

SALAD

- 1 large red beet
- 1 large orange beet
- 1 large yellow beet
- 3 tablespoons olive oil
- 1 tablespoon sea salt
- ½ tablespoon pepper
- ½ cup pea shoots
- 6–8 small edible flowers (optional)
- 2 tablespoons toasted sesame seeds

DRESSING

- ½ clove garlic, minced
- ½ teaspoon horseradish, grated
- 2 tablespoons champagne vinegar
- 1 tablespoon fresh lemon juice
- 1 tablespoon honey
- ¼ teaspoon salt
- ¼ teaspoon freshly ground black pepper

DIRECTIONS

Preheat oven to 350 degrees F.

Peel all beets. Place each beet on a sheet of foil big enough to wrap the beet. Drizzle 1 tablespoon of oil onto each beet and evenly season with salt and pepper. Wrap foil around the beets. Place the wrapped beets in the preheated oven and cook for 1 hour, or until fork-tender.

Mix all dressing ingredients in a container or jar with a top. Shake to combine.

Remove the beets from the oven and let cool. With a mandolin, thinly slice the beets. Arrange the beets by color in straight lines on a serving platter or individual plates. Pour a desired amount of dressing on top of the beets. Arrange the pea shoots, flowers and sesame seeds on top.

PER SERVING: SALAD: Calories: 151, Fat: 13g, Protein: 2.9g, Sodium: 1,372mg, Fiber: 2.6g, Carbohydrates: 7.8g, Sugar: 4.3g **DRESSING:** Calories: 24, Fat: 0g, Protein: 0.1g, Sodium: 114.5mg, Fiber: 0.1g, Carbohydrates: 6g, Sugar: 5.5g

HEARTY MUSHROOM AND SPINACH SOUP

Mushrooms help beef up this vegetable soup, making it the ultimate comfort dish.

INGREDIENTS

- 1 pound shiitake mushrooms
- 2 tablespoons olive oil
- 2 cloves garlic, minced
- 6 ounces fresh baby spinach
- 1 cup beef broth
- 5 cups vegetable broth
- 1 sprig thyme
- ½ teaspoon sea salt
- ½ teaspoon freshly ground black pepper

DIRECTIONS

SERVES 4

With a damp cloth or paper towel, wipe any dirt off the mushrooms before slicing them.

In a nonstick skillet coated with oil, cook the mushrooms over medium heat until softened and slightly brown, stirring frequently. Add the garlic and cook another minute.

Transfer the mushrooms and garlic to a soup pot and add the remaining ingredients. Bring the soup to a simmer. Over medium-low heat, let simmer 15 to 20 minutes. Remove the thyme sprig. Remove about half of the mushrooms and spinach and a couple of cups of liquid to a blender. Let cool slightly, then blend until smooth. Place back into the pot and simmer another 5 minutes before serving.

PER SERVING: Calories: 145, Fat: 7.1g, Protein: 7.2g, Sodium: 468mg, Fiber: 6.3g, Carbohydrates: 17g, Sugar: 3.1g

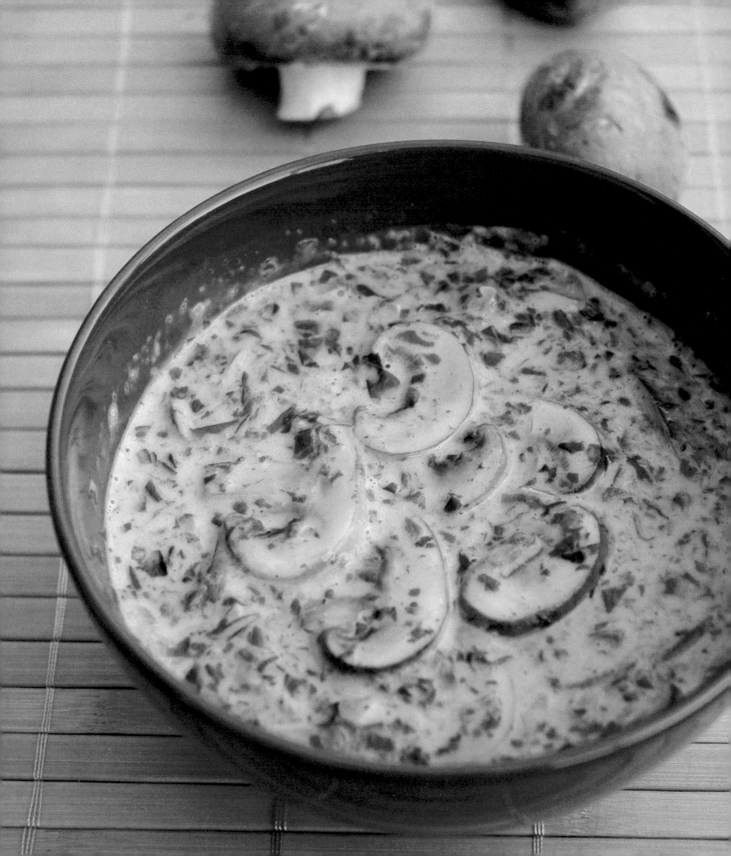

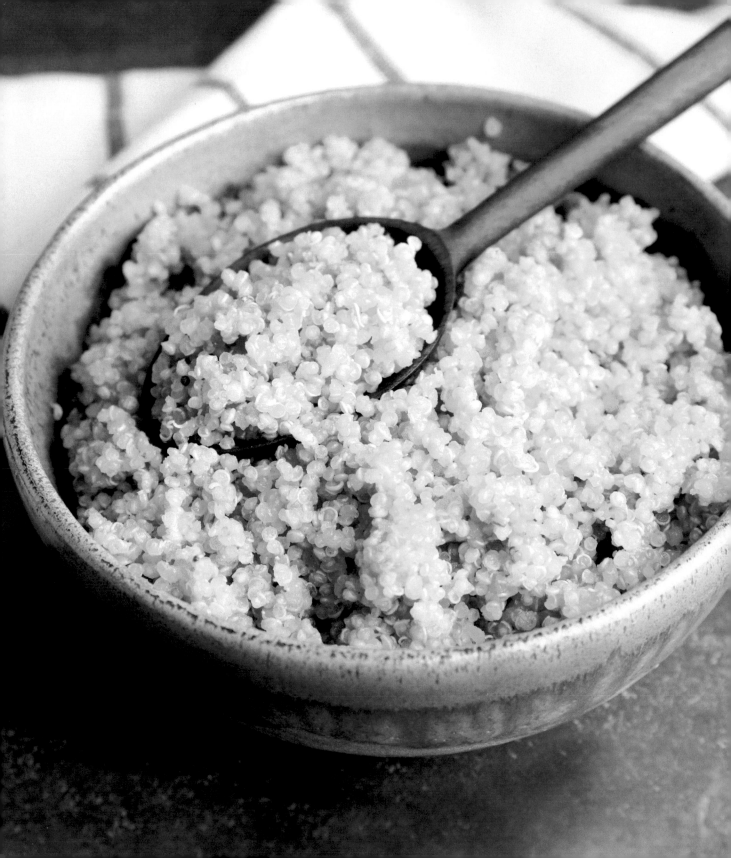

VEGETABLE QUINOA SALAD

This bright and flavorful salad is packed with protein and vitamins—you'll want to make it again and again!

| INGREDIENTS | DIRECTIONS | SERVES 4 |

SALAD

1¼ cups uncooked quinoa

2½ cups water

¼ teaspoon sea salt

4 cups Vegetable Chop (page 146)

DRESSING

½ lemon

6 tablespoons olive oil

1½ teaspoons white wine vinegar

1½ teaspoons mustard

¼ teaspoon salt

¼ teaspoon pepper

Combine the quinoa and salted water in a saucepan. Bring the mixture to a boil over medium-high and lower the heat to a simmer. Cook until the quinoa has absorbed all of the water, about 15 to 20 minutes. Remove the pot from the heat, cover and let the quinoa steam for 5 minutes. Remove the lid and fluff the quinoa with a fork.

Zest and juice the lemon into a container with a lid. Add the remaining dressing ingredients and shake until combined.

In a medium bowl, add the Vegetable Chop, cooked quinoa and dressing, then mix.

PER SERVING: SALAD: Calories: 320, Fat: 9.3g, Protein: 12g, Sodium: 252mg, Fiber: 7.4g, Carbohydrates: 49g, Sugar: 2.1g **DRESSING:** Calories: 183, Fat: 20.5g, Protein: 0.1g, Sodium: 140.5mg, Fiber: 0.1g, Carbohydrates: 0.5g, Sugar: 0.2g

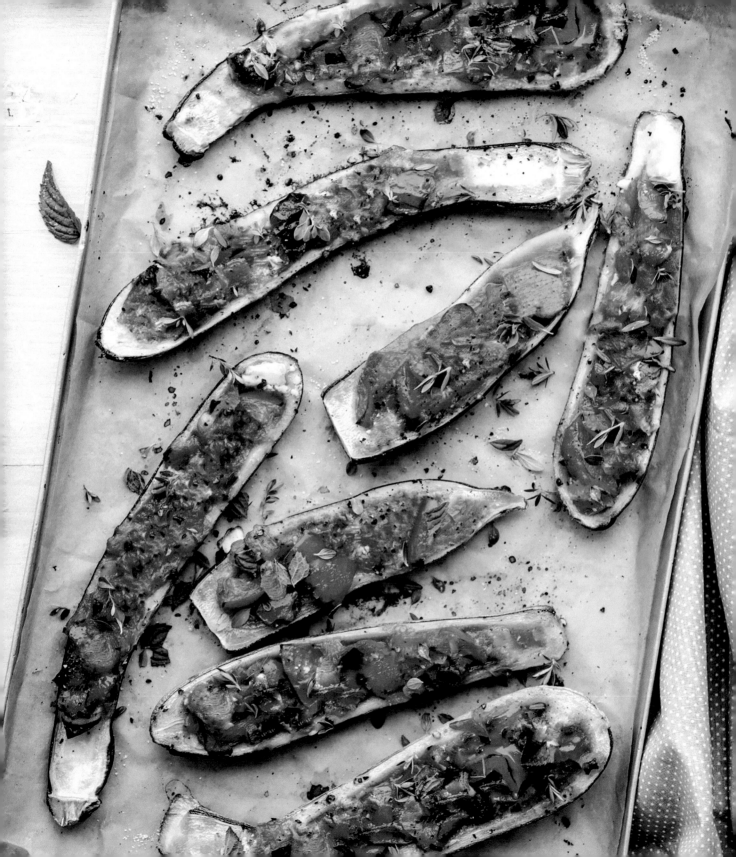

sides

LEAVE LOTS OF ROOM FOR THESE PRODUCE-PACKED SIDES.

Pan-Roasted Radishes **125**

Vegetable Fries with Lemon Garlic Gremolata **126**

Cauliflower Rice **129**

Red Rice Risotto **129**

Roasted Bok Choy **130**

Apple Cucumber Coleslaw **132**

Roasted Beets with Goat Cheese **133**

Five-Spice Butternut Squash Ribbons **134**

Sesame Ginger–Glazed Soba Noodles **134**

Cauliflower Fried Black Rice **136**

Beet Noodles with Red Pepper Pesto **137**

Roasted Tomato Zucchini Boats **138**

Dukkah Roasted Cauliflower **140**

Mexican Street Asparagus **141**

Pan-Fried Spicy Oyster Mushrooms **142**

Roasted and Mashed Turnips **145**

Vegetable Chop **146**

Roasted Squash with Tahini Sauce **147**

Sweet-and-Sour Swiss Chard **148**

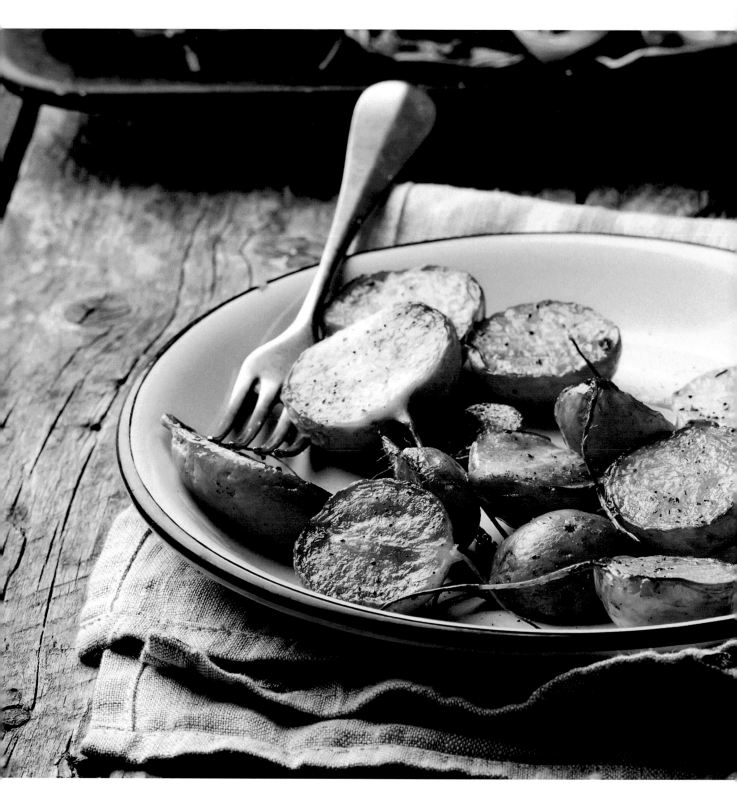

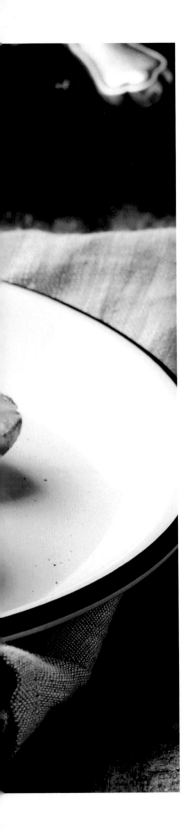

PAN-ROASTED RADISHES

Radishes are underutilized—these little root vegetables are full of flavor. Most times you will see radishes raw in salads, but pan roasting them mellows the peppery flavor and makes for a very different yet delicious dish.

INGREDIENTS	DIRECTIONS	SERVES 4

INGREDIENTS

- 2 pounds radishes
- 1 tablespoon olive oil
- ½ teaspoon salt
- Drizzle balsamic vinegar

DIRECTIONS

Cut the green tops off the radishes. Slice them into halves or quarters, making sure the pieces are roughly uniform in size.

In a large heavy-bottomed skillet, add the radishes and olive oil. Cook on medium-low heat, stirring often for about 20 minutes, or until the radishes are fork-tender. Place in a serving dish, season with salt and drizzle with balsamic vinegar and serve.

PER SERVING: Calories: 66, Fat: 3.6g, Protein: 1.5g, Sodium: 309mg, Fiber: 3.6g, Carbohydrates: 7.7g, Sugar: 4.2g

VEGETABLE FRIES WITH LEMON GARLIC GREMOLATA

These mixed vegetable "fries" are perfect for snacking, especially when they're served with a tasty gremolata.

INGREDIENTS

DIRECTIONS

SERVES 4

GREMOLATA

1 tablespoon olive oil

2 cloves garlic, minced

2 tablespoons fresh parsley, minced

¼ teaspoon fresh oregano, minced

¼ teaspoon sea salt

¼ teaspoon freshly ground black pepper

Zest of 1 lemon

FRIES

1 beet

1 bunch asparagus

2 cups green beans

2 tablespoons olive oil

½ tablespoon sea salt

½ tablespoon freshly ground black pepper

Preheat oven to 375 degrees F.

Add oil to a small nonstick frying pan over medium-low heat. Cook the garlic until just soft, about 2 minutes. Add the remaining gremolata ingredients to the pan and stir. Place the mixture into a bowl to cool.

Wash the beet, asparagus and beans. Peel the beet and cut it into a large julienne, like french fries. Place beets on a parchment-lined sheet pan. Drizzle with oil and season with salt and pepper. Mix to coat evenly.

Place in the preheated oven and cook for 20 minutes. Add asparagus and beans to the sheet pan, stirring to coat with oil and seasonings. Continue to cook for another 10 minutes, or until vegetables are fork-tender.

Place the fries onto serving plate, top with gremolata and serve.

PER SERVING: Calories: 140, Fat: 11g, Protein: 3.2g, Sodium: 615mg, Fiber: 4g, Carbohydrates: 11g, Sugar: 3.5g

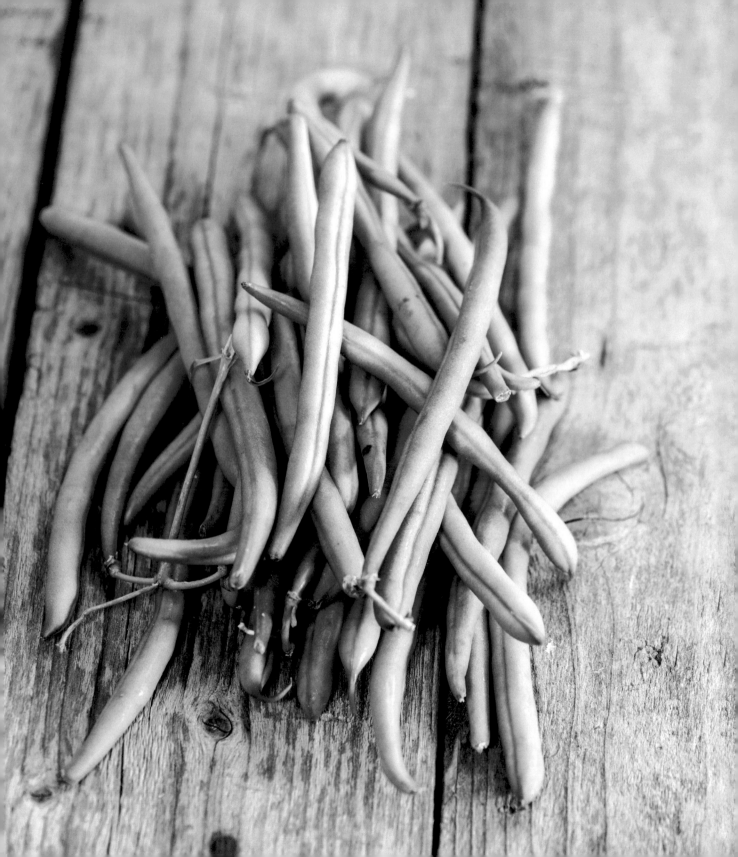

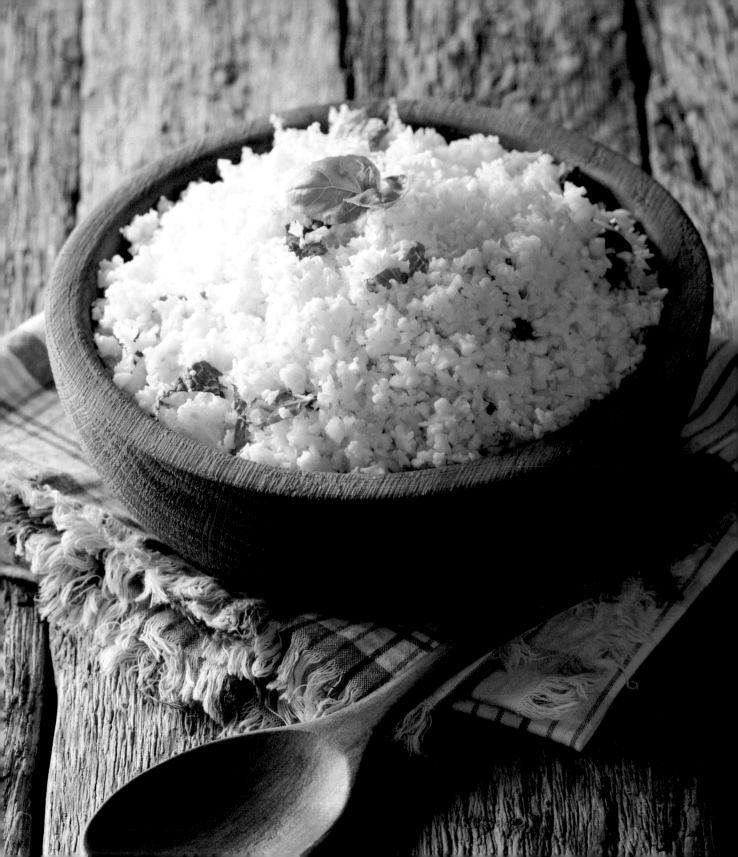

CAULIFLOWER RICE

Dress up this basic recipe with any herbs or seasonings you like—it's just as versatile as regular rice!

INGREDIENTS

- 1 head cauliflower
- 2 tablespoons olive oil
- ¼ teaspoon salt
- ¼ teaspoon freshly ground black pepper
- 1 tablespoon parsley, finely chopped

DIRECTIONS

SERVES 4

Cut the cauliflower into small pieces. Place the cauliflower in a food processor and pulse until broken down into rice-size pieces.

Heat the olive oil in a skillet with a lid over medium heat. Add the cauliflower, salt and pepper.

Cover the skillet and cook until heated through, about 3 to 5 minutes. Remove the lid and fluff the rice with a fork.

Garnish with parsley and serve.

PER SERVING: Calories: 113, Fat: 7.3g, Protein: 4g, Sodium: 283mg, Fiber: 4.3g, Carbohydrates: 11g, Sugar: 4g

RED RICE RISOTTO

If you're looking for a starchy side, this creamy and satisfying red rice risotto fits the bill.

INGREDIENTS

- 1¾ cups vegetable broth
- 1 tablespoon olive oil
- 1 large shallot, diced
- 2 cloves garlic, minced
- 1 cup red rice
- 1 tablespoon tomato paste
- ½ teaspoon sea salt
- ½ teaspoon freshly ground black pepper

DIRECTIONS

SERVES 4

In a small saucepan over medium heat, add the broth and bring to a simmer. Lower the heat to keep broth warm.

Add oil to a large skillet over medium heat. Cook the shallot and garlic for about 2 minutes. Add the rice and toast slightly, stirring frequently. Stir in the tomato paste and season with salt and pepper.

Slowly add one ladle of broth at a time until the rice is just covered. Let the broth cook into the rice, stirring almost constantly, before adding more broth. Continue until the rice is tender. Taste for seasoning and serve.

PER SERVING: Calories: 92, Fat: 4g, Protein: 2g, Sodium: 285mg, Fiber: 1.5g, Carbohydrates: 13g, Sugar: 2.5g

ROASTED BOK CHOY

Elevate any roasted vegetables—but especially this delicious Chinese cabbage—with this simple but oh-so-good dressing.

INGREDIENTS

DIRECTIONS

SERVES 4

- 8 bulbs of baby bok choy
- 1 tablespoon olive oil
- 2 tablespoons lemon
- 2 tablespoons honey
- ½ tablespoon apple cider vinegar
- ½ teaspoon sesame oil
- ½ teaspoon freshly ground black pepper
- ¼ teaspoon salt
- 1 teaspoon ginger, grated

Preheat oven to 350 degrees F.

Wash the bok choy and slice them into quarters. Place the bok choy on a parchment-lined sheet pan and drizzle with oil. Place them in the preheated oven and cook for 8 to 10 minutes, or until fork-tender.

In a small bowl, mix together the lemon, honey, vinegar, sesame oil, pepper, salt and grated ginger.

Place the roasted bok choy into a serving dish, mix in the dressing and serve.

PER SERVING: Calories: 86, Fat: 4g, Protein: 2g, Sodium: 330mg, Fiber: 2g, Carbohydrates: 13g, Sugar: 10g

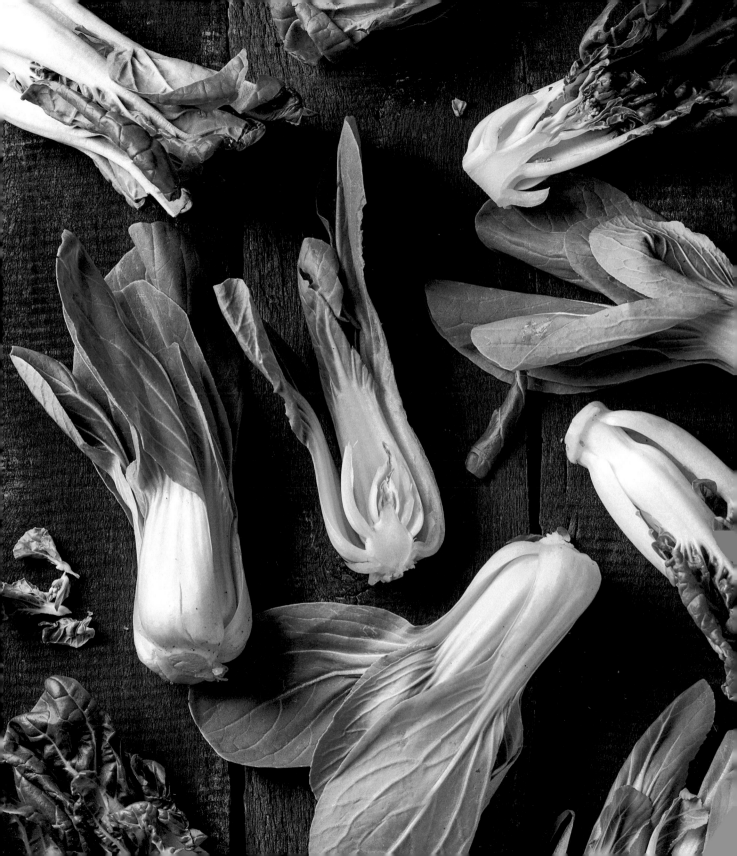

APPLE CUCUMBER COLESLAW

This coleslaw is delicious with just about anything, from sandwiches to tacos to salads.

INGREDIENTS

DIRECTIONS

- ½ small head cabbage, thinly sliced
- ½ English cucumber, julienned
- 3 honeycrisp apples, julienned
- ½ small red onion, minced
- ¼ cup apple cider vinegar
- 1 tablespoon lemon juice
- 2 tablespoons olive oil
- ½ teaspoon salt
- ½ teaspoon freshly ground black pepper
- 1 tablespoon fresh dill, chopped
- 1 teaspoon fresh parsley, chopped
- ½ teaspoon celery seed
- ½ jalapeño pepper, seeded and julienned

Add all ingredients to a large bowl and mix well. Refrigerate for an hour, or until cold.

PER SERVING: Calories: 115, Fat: 4.7g, Protein: 1.5g, Sodium: 173mg, Fiber: 4.7g, Carbohydrates: 19g, Sugar: 12g

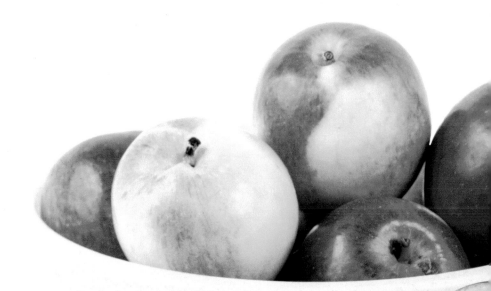

ROASTED BEETS WITH GOAT CHEESE

Goat cheese and beets go together wonderfully. The earthiness of the beets and the tangy saltiness from the cheese bring the perfect balance to this dish.

INGREDIENTS   **DIRECTIONS**   SERVES 4

- 1 large red beet
- 1 large orange beet
- 1 large yellow beet
- 2 tablespoons olive oil
- 1 tablespoon salt
- 1 tablespoon freshly ground black pepper
- 3 ounces goat cheese

Preheat oven to 400 degrees F.

Peel the beets. Place each beet on a sheet of foil big enough to wrap the beet. Drizzle each with oil and season with an even amount of salt and pepper. Close the foil tight on top and place in a preheated oven for 1 hour, or until the beets are fork-tender.

Take the beets out of the foil. Cut them in quarters (or halves if using smaller beets), making sure they are roughly uniform in size. Place in a serving dish, top with the crumbled goat cheese and serve.

PER SERVING: Calories: 147, Fat: 11g, Protein: 5.1g, Sodium: 1,466mg, Fiber: 2.1g, Carbohydrates: 7g, Sugar: 4.4g

FIVE-SPICE BUTTERNUT SQUASH RIBBONS

Using a mandolin or vegetable peeler to turn the squash
into ribbons makes this side dish a show-stopper.

INGREDIENTS

- 1 butternut squash
- 2 tablespoons olive oil
- 1 teaspoon five-spice
- 1 teaspoon sea salt
- 1 teaspoon freshly ground black pepper
- 2 tablespoons salted pepitas
- 1 teaspoon cayenne

DIRECTIONS   **SERVES 4**

Peel and deseed the squash. With a vegetable peeler or mandolin slicer, thinly slice the squash into ribbon slices.

Add olive oil to a large sauté pan and heat over medium. Add the squash ribbons, five-spice, salt and pepper. Cook the squash for 5 minutes, or until vegetables are crisp-tender.

Meanwhile, toast the pepitas in a small frying pan until lightly toasted. Sprinkle the pepitas with cayenne.

Place the sautéed squash on a serving plate, top with pepitas and serve.

PER SERVING: Calories: 218, Fat: 7.4g, Protein: 3.7g, Sodium: 454mg, Fiber: 7g, Carbohydrates: 40g, Sugar: 7.5g

SESAME GINGER-GLAZED SOBA NOODLES

Soba noodles are made of buckwheat, which is, despite the name, not wheat at all but a cousin of rhubarb. They're very healthy and especially delicious when covered in this sesame ginger glaze.

INGREDIENTS

- 12 ounces soba noodles
- 1 tablespoon soy sauce
- 1 tablespoon honey
- 1 teaspoon lime juice
- 1 teaspoon fresh ginger, grated
- 1 teaspoon minced garlic
- 2 teaspoons sesame seeds, toasted

DIRECTIONS   **SERVES 4**

In a large pot filled with boiling water, cook the soba noodles for 4 to 5 minutes, or until al dente. Turn off the heat, drain the noodles and return them to the pot.

In a small bowl, mix together the soy sauce, honey, lime juice, ginger, garlic and toasted sesame seeds. Add the mixture to the pot with noodles and toss to coat all of the noodles.

PER SERVING: Calories: 115, Fat: 0.9g, Protein: 5.2g, Sodium: 303mg, Fiber: 0.3g, Carbohydrates: 24g, Sugar: 4.1g

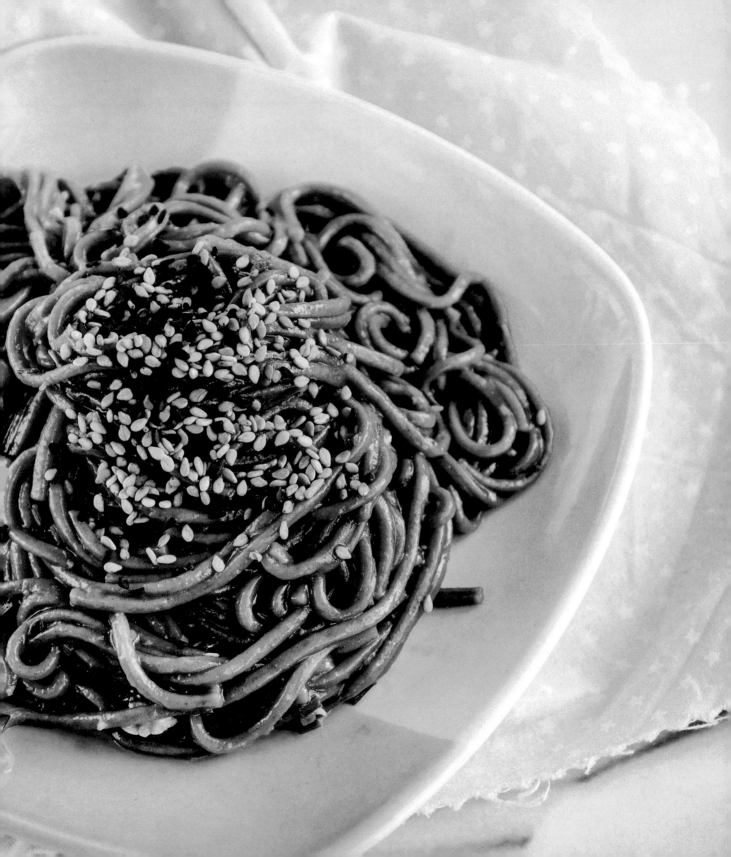

CAULIFLOWER FRIED BLACK RICE

Also known as forbidden rice, black rice is a healthier alternative to white rice. It can be used in all the same ways and is especially tasty in this spin on classic fried rice.

INGREDIENTS

- 1 cup black rice
- 2 eggs
- 1 tablespoon olive oil
- 1½ cups shaved Brussels sprouts
- ½ red onion, diced
- ½ red bell pepper, diced
- 2 cloves garlic, diced
- 3 cups prepared Cauliflower Rice (page 129)
- 1 teaspoon sea salt
- 1 teaspoon freshly ground black pepper

DIRECTIONS

SERVES 4

Rinse the black rice and cook according to package instructions. Let cool.

In a small bowl, mix together the eggs and set aside.

In a large nonstick frying pan, cast-iron pan or wok on medium heat, add oil and cook the Brussels sprouts, onion and pepper until just tender. Stir in garlic.

Add both the black rice and the cauliflower rice to the pan, increase the heat to high and cook for about 4 minutes, stirring every minute and adding more oil if needed. Make a well in the middle of the rice and add the eggs, stirring to scramble. Once the eggs are cooked, mix them into the rice and season with salt and pepper.

PER SERVING: Calories: 153, Fat: 6.5g, Protein: 7.8g, Sodium: 509mg, Fiber: 4.4g, Carbohydrates: 18g, Sugar: 4.4g

BEET NOODLES WITH RED PEPPER PESTO

This nutritional powerhouse of a side dish boasts vibrant colors
and flavors—you'll find yourself having seconds!

| INGREDIENTS | DIRECTIONS | SERVES 4 |

PESTO

- 1 red bell pepper
- ¼ cup pine nuts
- 2 cloves garlic
- ½ cup olive oil
- 1 tablespoon horseradish
- ½ teaspoon sea salt

NOODLES

- 3 large red beets
- 1 tablespoon olive oil
- ½ teaspoon salt
- ½ teaspoon freshly ground black pepper

On an open flame from a gas stove or grill, roast the pepper until charred and blistered. Let the pepper sit to cool, then remove the skin, stem and seeds.

Lightly toast the pine nuts in a small saucepan over medium-low heat for about 3 minutes.

Place all pesto ingredients in a food processor and blend until smooth.

Cut the beets with a spiralizer. Heat a nonstick pan over medium with the oil. Add the beets and cook for 5 to 7 minutes, or until fork-tender, stirring occasionally.

Place the beets into a bowl, top with the pesto and mix to combine.

PER SERVING: Calories: 362, Fat: 36g, Protein: 2.4g, Sodium: 514mg, Fiber: 2.7g, Carbohydrates: 9.4g, Sugar: 5.8g

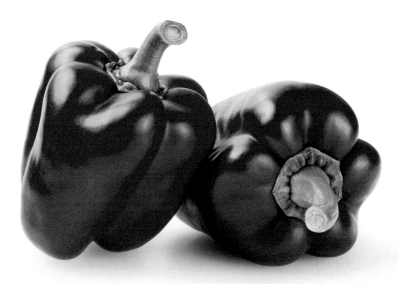

ROASTED TOMATO ZUCCHINI BOATS

Roasted tomatoes and fresh basil take these zucchini boats in a decidedly Italian direction, but you can fill them with any roasted veggies and spice mix you like.

INGREDIENTS

DIRECTIONS

SERVES 4

- 2 medium zucchinis
- 2 pints grape or cherry tomatoes, chopped
- 1 small bunch fresh basil leaves, torn
- 1 onion, sliced
- 2 cloves garlic, minced
- 1 teaspoon salt
- 1 teaspoon freshly ground black pepper
- 3 tablespoons olive oil

Preheat oven to 375 degrees F.

Slice the zucchinis in half lengthwise, scoop out the seeds. Fill each zucchini evenly with the tomatoes, basil, onions and garlic and season with salt and pepper. Drizzle oil on top of each and place on a parchment-lined sheet pan.

Place in the preheated oven. Cook for about 20 minutes, or until the zucchini is fork-tender.

PER SERVING: Calories: 155, Fat: 10g, Protein: 3.7g, Sodium: 460mg, Fiber: 3.8g, Carbohydrates: 13g, Sugar: 6g

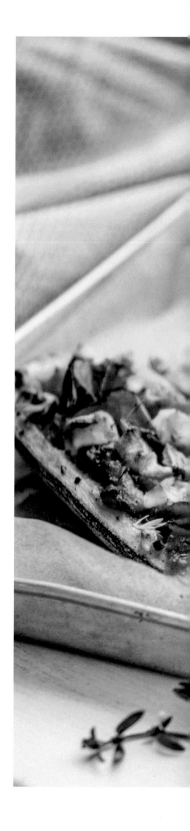

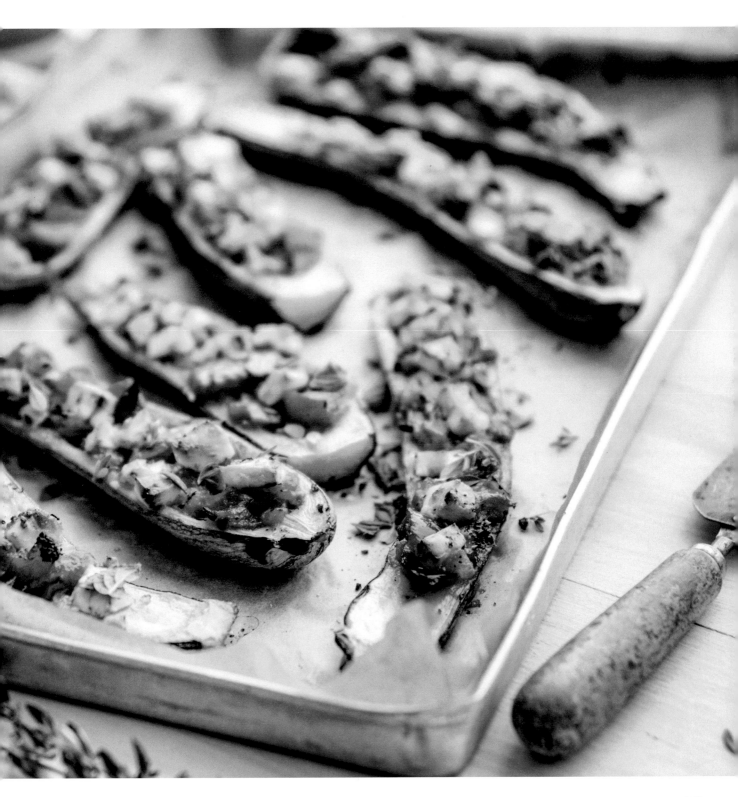

DUKKAH ROASTED CAULIFLOWER

Use dukkah to turn cauliflower or any other vegetable into your favorite new side dish.

INGREDIENTS **DIRECTIONS** SERVES 4

CAULIFLOWER

1 head cauliflower

1 tablespoon olive oil

DUKKAH

2 tablespoons sesame seeds

¼ cup raw pistachios

¼ cup blanched almonds

¼ cup coriander seeds

1½ teaspoons cumin seeds

1 teaspoon red chili powder

¼ teaspoon sea salt

⅛ teaspoon freshly ground black pepper

Preheat oven to 350 degrees F.

Wash the cauliflower and trim off the leafy ends and extra stalk. Place the cauliflower stem-side down on a parchment-lined sheet pan. Brush the cauliflower with oil.

In a large non-stick frying pan on medium heat, toast sesame seeds until golden brown, about 3 to 4 minutes. Remove and set aside. In the same pan, toast pistachios and almonds until slightly toasted, about 3 minutes. Remove and set aside. In the same pan, toast coriander and cumin seeds until slightly toasted, about 2 minutes. In a food processor, add all dukkah ingredients except sesame seeds and pulse the mixture together until coarsely ground. Stir in sesame seeds.

Sprinkle 2 tablespoons dukkah seasoning onto the cauliflower, using your hands to make sure it adheres to the sides. Save the rest of the dukkah for future uses.

Place in a preheated oven on the middle rack and cook for about 1 hour, or until cauliflower is fork-tender, covering with foil if it starts to get too brown.

PER SERVING: Calories: 227, Fat: 17g, Protein: 8g, Sodium: 287mg, Fiber: 8g, Carbohydrates: 17g, Sugar: 4.7g

MEXICAN STREET ASPARAGUS

Swap in asparagus for corn to enjoy this tasty Mexican side while staying pegan.

INGREDIENTS	DIRECTIONS	SERVES 4

INGREDIENTS

- 2 bunches asparagus
- 1 tablespoon olive oil
- ½ teaspoon salt
- ½ cup Avocado Crema (page 163)
- 1 clove garlic, minced
- ¼ teaspoon ground chipotle pepper
- 2 teaspoons lime juice
- Zest of ½ lime, plus extra for garnish
- Cilantro, for garnish

DIRECTIONS

Preheat the grill on medium heat.

Wash the asparagus and remove the woody ends by bending each stalk and letting it naturally break. Brush with olive oil and season with salt.

In a bowl, mix together the Avocado Crema, garlic, chipotle pepper, lime juice and zest.

Place the asparagus on a hot grill and cook for 2 to 4 minutes, turning once during cooking. Remove the asparagus from the heat, place on a serving platter and top with sauce. Garnish with lime zest and cilantro.

PER SERVING: Calories: 123, Fat: 8.7g, Protein: 4.4g, Sodium: 670mg, Fiber: 4.9g, Carbohydrates: 8.4g, Sugar: 1.9g

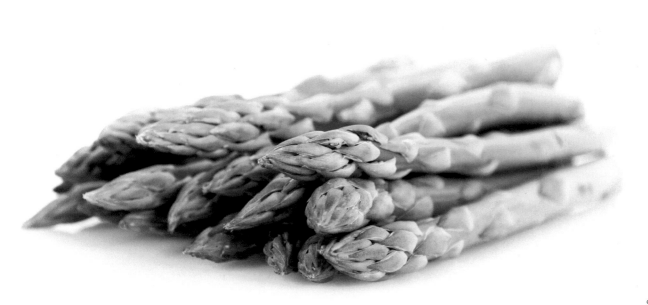

PAN-FRIED SPICY OYSTER MUSHROOMS

If you like it hot, this is the side dish for you! If you're less daring,
dial back the red pepper flakes in this recipe.

INGREDIENTS

DIRECTIONS

SERVES 2-4

- 1½ pounds oyster mushrooms
- 2 tablespoons olive oil
- ½ cup sliced leeks, white and light green parts only
- 2 cloves garlic, sliced
- ½ teaspoon sea salt
- ½ teaspoon freshly ground black pepper
- ¼ cup fresh parsley, chopped
- 1 tablespoon red pepper flakes

Wipe any debris and dirt from the mushrooms with a damp cloth or paper towel. Cut the mushrooms into bite-size pieces.

Place the oil in a nonstick pan and heat over medium. Cook the mushrooms undisturbed for 3 to 4 minutes. Stir and cook for 3 to 4 more minutes, then stir in the leeks and continue to cook for 2 to 3 minutes. Add the garlic, season with salt, pepper, parsley and red pepper flakes and continue to cook for another minute. Place the mushroom mixture into a bowl and serve.

PER SERVING: Calories: 125, Fat: 7.5g, Protein: 5.8g, Sodium: 253mg,
Fiber: 4g, Carbohydrates: 12g, Sugar: 2.3g

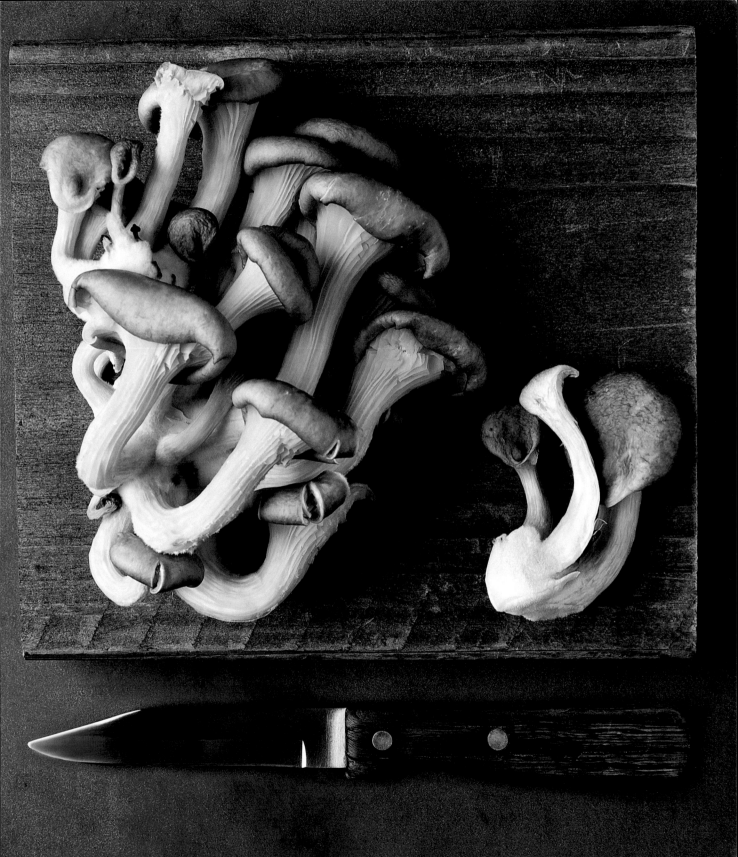

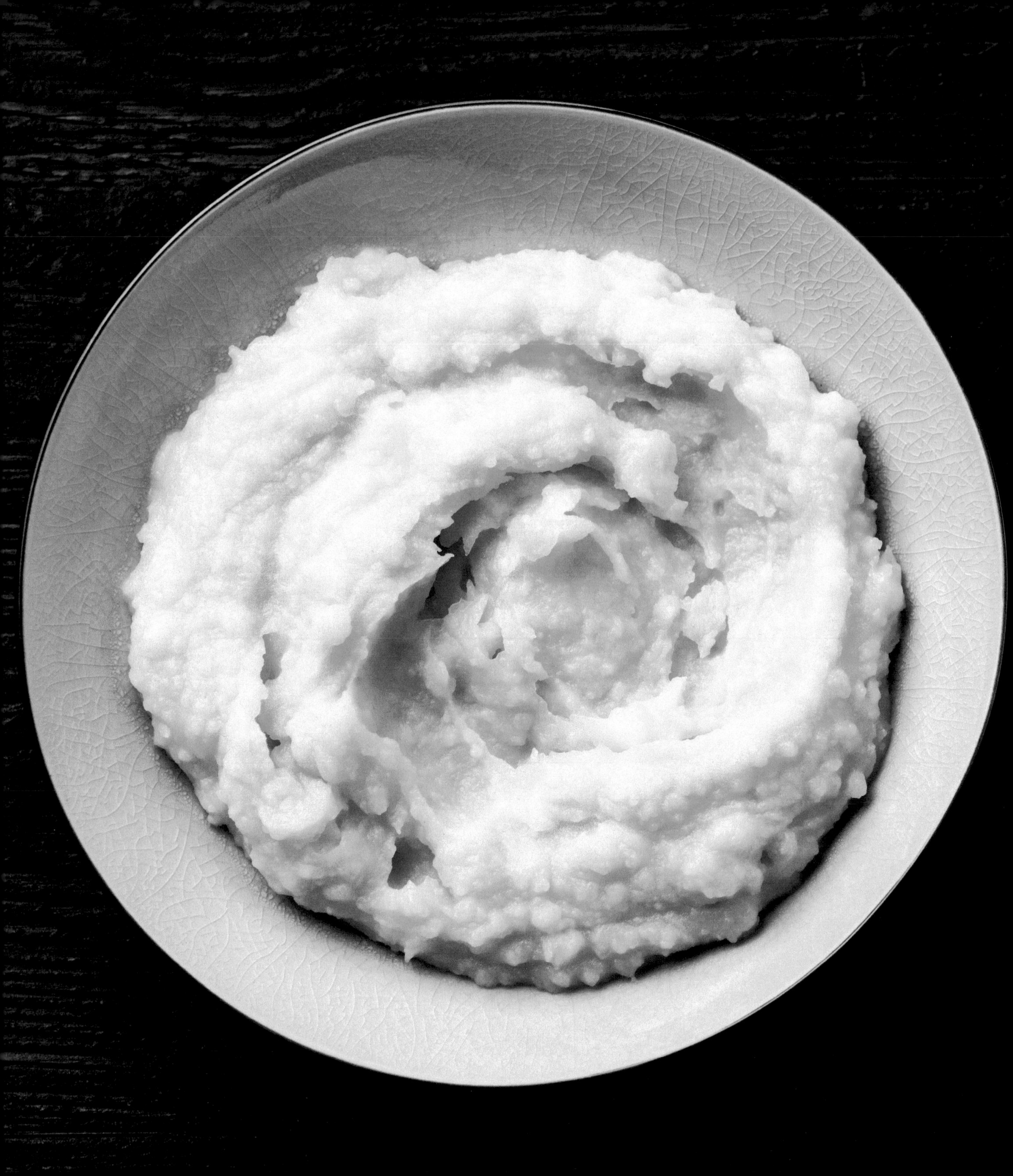

ROASTED AND MASHED TURNIPS

These mashed turnips are a great alternative to mashed potatoes. Adding horseradish gives this side just the right texture and the perfect amount of spice.

INGREDIENTS	DIRECTIONS	SERVES 4

INGREDIENTS

- 1 large turnip
- 1 tablespoon olive oil
- 1 teaspoon sea salt, divided
- 1 teaspoon freshly ground black pepper, divided
- 1 cup almond milk
- 2 tablespoons horseradish
- 3 tablespoons fresh chives, diced

DIRECTIONS

Preheat oven to 350 degrees F.

Peel and cut the turnip into 1-inch pieces. Place on a parchment-lined cookie sheet. Drizzle with olive oil and season with ½ teaspoon salt and pepper. Mix to coat evenly. Place the turnips in oven. Cook for 20 to 30 minutes, or until the turnips are fork-tender.

In a large pot over medium heat, add the remaining salt, pepper, milk and horseradish and bring to a gentle simmer.

Remove from heat and add in the roasted turnips. With a blender, mixer or handheld masher, mash the turnips until smooth, adding more milk if necessary. Fold in the chives and serve.

PER SERVING: Calories: 54, Fat: 4g, Protein: 0.8g, Sodium: 531mg, Fiber: 1.4g, Carbohydrates: 4g, Sugar: 2.4g

VEGETABLE CHOP

If you're not getting enough cruciferous vegetables turn to this dish! It's the perfect base for proteins or could even be served up for breakfast with a fried egg on top.

INGREDIENTS

- 1 head broccoli
- 3 cups Brussels sprouts
- 3 tablespoons olive oil, divided
- ½ teaspoon sea salt
- ½ teaspoon freshly ground black pepper
- 1 leek

DIRECTIONS

Preheat oven to 350 degrees F.

Wash the broccoli and Brussels sprouts. Cut the broccoli into florets. Trim the ends off the Brussels sprouts and cut them in half. Place the Brussels sprouts and broccoli on a parchment-lined cookie sheet. Drizzle with 2 tablespoons oil, season with salt and pepper and mix to evenly coat. Cook in the preheated oven for 15 to 20 minutes, or until the vegetables are fork-tender.

Cut the leek in half lengthwise, keeping the root attached. Run the leek under cold water and wash away any sand between the leaves. Cut off the root and slice the white and light-green parts of the leek. In a small saucepan over medium heat, add the remaining tablespoon of oil and sauté the leeks until just tender. Remove from the pan and let cool.

Using a large cutting board, chop the roasted vegetables and leeks, then mix them together to a hash-like consistency.

SERVES 4

PER SERVING: Calories: 170, Fat: 11g, Protein: 5.8g, Sodium: 279mg, Fiber: 5.9g, Carbohydrates: 17g, Sugar: 4.2g

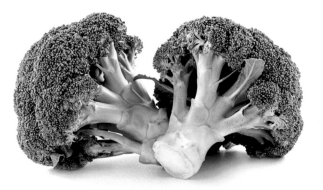

ROASTED SQUASH WITH TAHINI SAUCE

Serving hot squash with this creamy, garlicky and cool tahini sauce makes for a perfect balance of flavors. Save any extra sauce—it makes for a great dip with other vegetables too.

INGREDIENTS | DIRECTIONS | SERVES 4

SQUASH

- 1 kabocha squash
- 1 tablespoon olive oil
- ½ teaspoon sea salt
- ½ teaspoon freshly ground black pepper

SAUCE

- ¼ cup rice wine vinegar
- ¼ cup fresh lemon juice
- ½ cup tahini
- ¼ cup olive oil
- 1 clove garlic, minced
- ½ teaspoon sea salt
- ½ teaspoon freshly ground black pepper

Preheat oven to 375 degrees F.

Wash the squash and cut off the ends. Slice the squash into 1½-inch rounds.

Place the cut squash on a parchment-lined sheet pan. Drizzle the squash with oil and season with salt and pepper. Place in the preheated oven and cook for about 40 minutes, or until the squash is fork-tender.

Place all sauce ingredients in a blender and blend until smooth, adding water if the sauce is too thick.

Take the squash out of the oven and place it on a serving platter. Drizzle with sauce and serve.

PER SERVING: Calories: 344, Fat: 33g, Protein: 5.6g, Sodium: 475mg, Fiber: 3.6g, Carbohydrates: 11g, Sugar: 1.7g

SWEET-AND-SOUR SWISS CHARD

This sweet-and-sour dressing goes great with Swiss chard and other leafy greens, such as spinach, kale or even bok choy.

INGREDIENTS

- 2 large bunches of Swiss chard
- 2 tablespoons olive oil
- 2 cloves garlic, sliced
- ½ cup sherry vinegar
- 1 tablespoon honey
- ½ teaspoon salt
- ½ teaspoon freshly ground black pepper

DIRECTIONS

SERVES 4

Clean and dry the Swiss chard leaves. Cut out the stems and cut in a large chiffonade by placing the leaves on top of each other, rolling them together, then cutting down about every ¾ inch to make ribbons.

Place the Swiss chard into a large skillet with oil over medium heat. Cook the Swiss chard for 3 to 4 minutes, or until wilted. Add the garlic and cook for another minute. Add in the vinegar, honey, salt and pepper and cook for another minute. Place in a serving dish and serve.

PER SERVING: Calories: 88, Fat: 6.8g, Protein: 0.6g, Sodium: 303mg, Fiber: 0.6g, Carbohydrates: 10g, Sugar: 8.4g

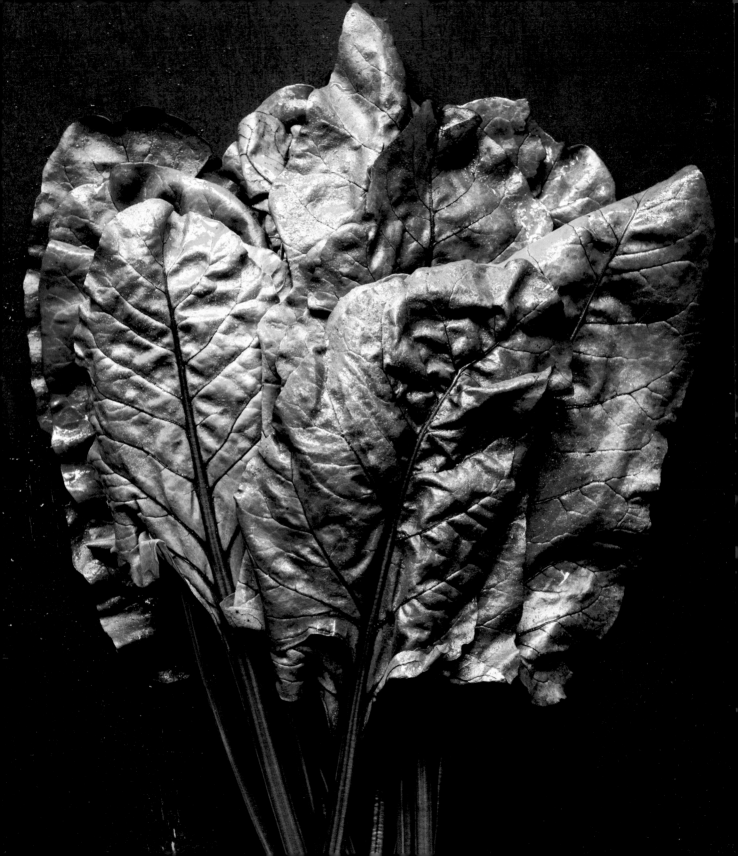

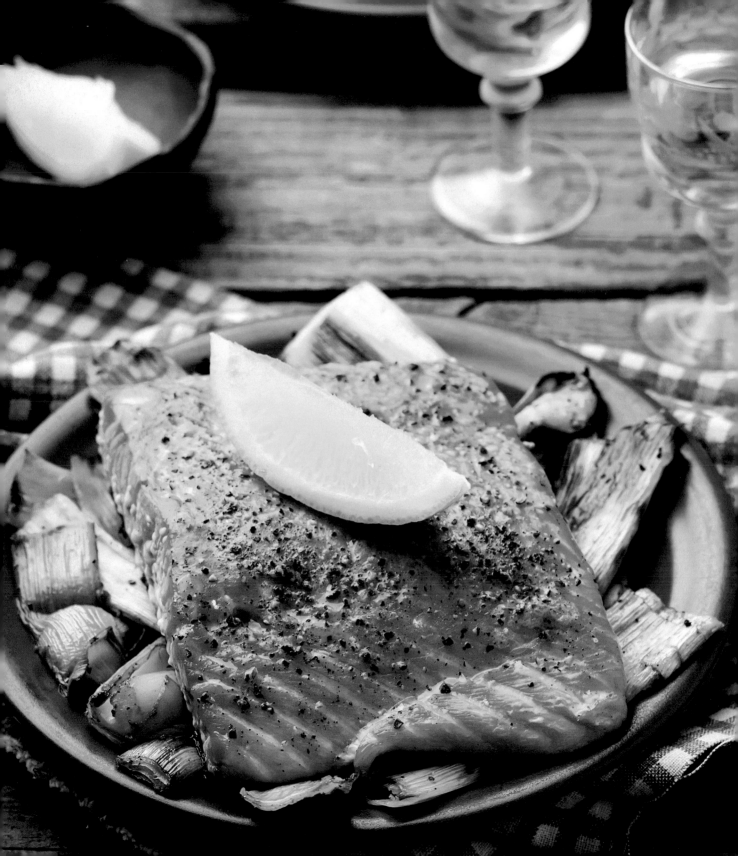

mains

WHIP UP AN EASY AND DELICIOUS LUNCH OR DINNER.

Braised Short Ribs 153

Blackberry Lamb Chop 154

Fettuccine Alfredo 155

Roasted Garlic and
Herb Millet Polenta 157

Hot Chicken Wings Piccata 158

Salmon Salad Sliders 159

Asian Skillet Salmon 160

Vegetable and Mussels Bowl 160

Buffalo Cauliflower
Lettuce Cups 162

Stuffed Poblano Peppers 163

Quinoa and Sweet Potato Burger 165

Orange Pepper Pesto-Stuffed
Roasted Cabbage Steaks 166

Mushroom Stew 167

Skillet Braised Salmon
and Vegetables 169

Mediterranean Vegetable
Shrimp Scampi 170

Chicken and Pineapple
Skewers 171

Slow Cooker Pulled Pork 172

Stuffed Meatloaf 172

Seared Scallops over
Green Beans, Tomatoes
and Microgreens 174

Slow Cooker Chicken Cacciatore 175

Stuffed Eggplant 176

Shrimp Dinner Pockets 178

Soba Noodles and Clam Sauce 179

Thai Orange Ginger
Baby Back Ribs 181

Artisan Tomato Sandwich with
Healthy Sandwich Spread 182

Beef and Broccoli 183

Swedish Meatballs 184

Grilled Pork Tenderloin
Chops with Plum Sauce 186

Sweet Potato Black Bean Chili 187

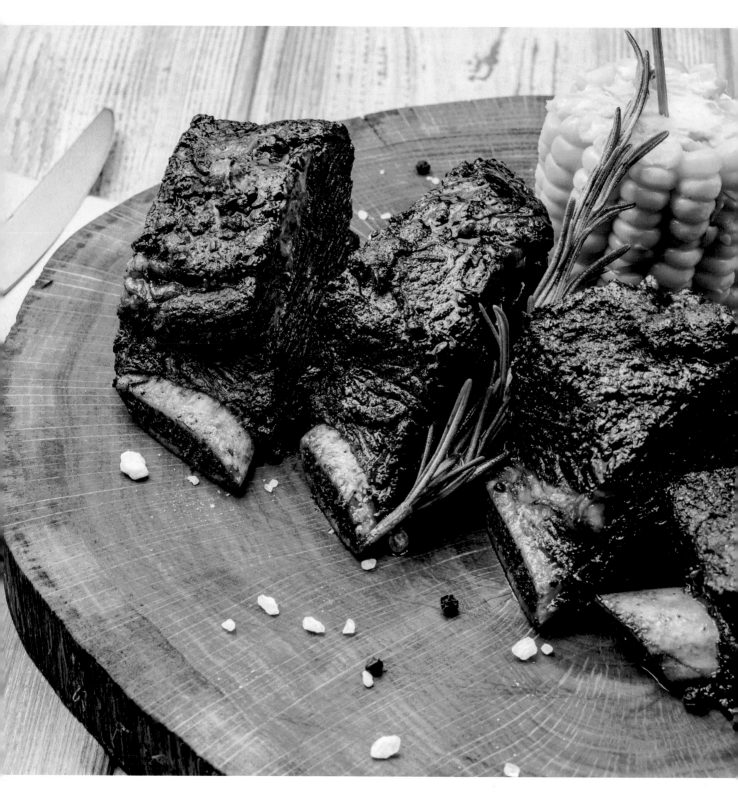

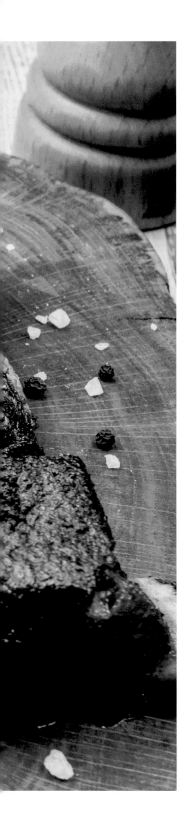

BRAISED SHORT RIBS

Braised beef is both a comfort food and perfect for a pegan diet—the flavorful ribs come with little meat on them, leaving room for lots of vegetables on your plate.

INGREDIENTS	DIRECTIONS	SERVES 4

INGREDIENTS

- 3 pounds bone-in short ribs
- 1 teaspoon sea salt
- 1 teaspoon freshly ground black pepper
- 3 tablespoons olive oil
- 3 cups beef broth, plus more as needed
- ½ teaspoon fresh thyme leaves
- ¼ teaspoon fresh rosemary
- 2 tablespoons fresh parsley, chopped

DIRECTIONS

Season the short ribs with salt and pepper.

Heat a large Dutch oven over medium-high. Add oil and sear all sides of the meat until browned. You may need to sear in batches in order to not crowd the meat. Place all of the meat back into the Dutch oven and add the broth, thyme and rosemary. Add more broth if the meat is not covered. Lower the heat to a simmer, place the lid on and simmer for 2½ to 3 hours. Remove the ribs from the pot and set aside. Continue to simmer until the sauce is reduced by ¼. Place the short ribs on the serving dish, drizzle with the sauce, garnish with parsley and serve.

PER SERVING: Calories: 900, Fat: 72g, Protein: 61g, Sodium: 1,328mg, Fiber: 0g, Carbohydrates: 0.8g, Sugar: 0.8g

BLACKBERRY LAMB CHOP

Fruit and lamb is a classic pairing: the light sweetness of the fruit cuts into the earthiness of the lamb. If you'd like, serve this dish over Vegetable Chop (page 146).

INGREDIENTS

DIRECTIONS

SERVES 4

BLACKBERRY SAUCE

- 1 tablespoon olive oil
- ½ small shallot, diced
- 3 cloves garlic
- ½ cup chicken broth
- 1 pint fresh blackberries
- 1 teaspoon fresh thyme
- 2 anchovies

LAMB CHOPS

- 4 (4-ounce) lamb chops
- ½ teaspoon salt
- ½ teaspoon freshly ground black pepper

Heat a medium saucepan over medium-low. Add the oil, shallots and garlic. Cook until tender. Add in the remaining blackberry sauce ingredients. Simmer for 10 minutes, or until the anchovies are melted and the sauce has reduced by ¼. Strain the sauce with a small mesh colander.

Preheat the grill to medium-high heat.

Season the lamb chops with salt and pepper. Brush the blackberry sauce on both sides of each chop. Cook the lamb chops on the preheated grill for about 2 minutes on each side, or to an internal temperature of 130 degrees F. Lay a piece of foil over the chops and let rest for 5 to 7 minutes.

Serve with the remaining sauce on the side.

PER SERVING: Calories: 417, Fat: 33g, Protein: 20g, Sodium: 336mg, Fiber: 4g, Carbohydrates: 8.8g, Sugar: 4.1g

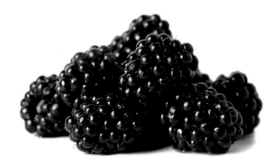

FETTUCCINE ALFREDO

Butternut squash noodles are a healthy alternative to traditional pastas—their firmness makes for a hearty, pasta-like bite. As a bonus, this delicious dairy-free cheese sauce can be used on any recipe including tacos, pizza and more.

INGREDIENTS	DIRECTIONS	SERVES 4

INGREDIENTS

GRATED CHEESE

- ¾ cup raw cashews
- 2 tablespoons nutritional yeast
- ½ teaspoon sea salt
- ½ teaspoon ground white pepper
- ¼ teaspoon onion powder

CHEESE SAUCE

- 5 cups cashews
- 1 clove garlic, minced
- 3 tablespoons nutritional yeast
- 1 tablespoon lemon juice
- 1 teaspoon sea salt
- ½ teaspoon mustard powder
- Water or almond milk

SQUASH NOODLES

- 1 large butternut squash
- 2 tablespoons olive oil
- 1 tablespoon sea salt

DIRECTIONS

In a food processor, add all grated cheese ingredients and pulse until you reach a grated cheese consistency. Set aside.

Soak the cashews in water for 2 to 4 hours. Drain.

Add the cashews, garlic, yeast, lemon juice, salt and mustard to a high-powered blender and purée, adding just enough water while you are blending to get a smooth consistency.

Preheat oven to 375 degrees F.

Cut the ends off the squash and cut in half lengthwise, scrape out the seeds and peel the skin. Cut into smaller pieces that can fit in a spiralizer. With a spiralizer fitted with a large noodle cutter, spiralize the squash.

Place the cut squash on a parchment-lined sheet pan with oil and season with salt. Place in the preheated oven and cook for 8 to 10 minutes, or until softened with some bite in the middle (al dente).

Mix together the squash and cheese sauce. Add in the grated cheese, toss again to mix and serve.

PER SERVING: Calories: 1,563, Fat: 116g, Protein: 46g, Sodium: 2,045mg, Fiber: 14g, Carbohydrates: 106g, Sugar: 19g

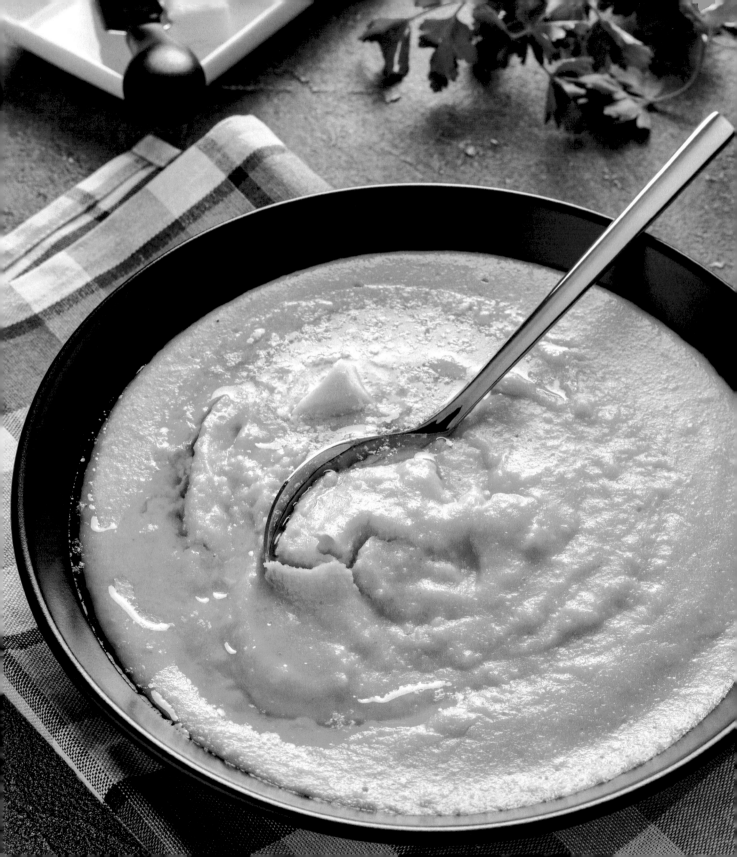

ROASTED GARLIC AND HERB MILLET POLENTA

There is nothing more comforting than a delicious bowl of polenta—it's the perfect base for stews and braises or simply topped with roast vegetables.

INGREDIENTS

- 1 small head garlic
- ½ tablespoon olive oil
- ¾ cup millet
- 4 cups vegetable broth
- 1 tablespoon fresh parsley, chopped
- 1 tablespoon fresh basil, chopped
- ½ teaspoon fresh rosemary, minced
- ½ teaspoon sea salt
- ¼ teaspoon freshly ground black pepper

DIRECTIONS

SERVES 4

Preheat oven to 375 degrees F.

Cut the top off of the garlic, place on foil and drizzle with oil. Wrap the foil around the garlic and bake until tender, about 35 to 45 minutes.

With a food processor, pulse the millet until about half of the grains are broken.

In a medium saucepan over medium heat, add the broth and bring to a boil. Slowly whisk in the millet. Add the roasted garlic and herbs and season with salt and pepper. Lower the heat to a simmer and cook, stirring often, for 40 to 45 minutes, or until creamy and grain is soft.

PER SERVING: Calories: 182, Fat: 3.3g, Protein: 5.2g, Sodium: 582mg, Fiber: 4.2g, Carbohydrates: 32g, Sugar: 2g

HOT CHICKEN WINGS PICCATA

These hot wings are a perfect party appetizer, but they also make for a fun dinner served with a salad.

INGREDIENTS

2 pounds chicken wings

2 tablespoons olive oil

2 tablespoons horseradish

2 lemons, juice and zest

¼ cup capers

¼ teaspoon salt

¼ teaspoon pepper

Chicken broth

Parsley, chopped, for garnish

DIRECTIONS

SERVES 4-6

Preheat oven to 375 degrees F.

Cut the wings in three sections. Discard the wing tips or save for stock.

In a blender, pulse the oil, horseradish, lemon juice, lemon zest, capers, salt and pepper together, adding in enough chicken broth to make a chunky sauce with the consistency of ketchup.

Place the wings on a parchment-lined sheet pan. Brush an even layer of sauce onto each chicken wing. Place in the preheated oven and bake until the chicken is cooked through, about 15 to 20 minutes.

Remove the wings from the oven, place on serving plate and garnish with parsley. Serve with leftover sauce.

PER SERVING: Calories: 645, Fat: 45g, Protein: 54g, Sodium: 474mg, Fiber: 0.3g, Carbohydrates: 2.5g, Sugar: 1.2g

SALMON SALAD SLIDERS

These salmon sliders are a perfect summertime meal—they're simple yet tasty and easy enough to make for a crowd.

INGREDIENTS	DIRECTIONS	SERVES 4

SALAD

3 avocados

½ lemon, juiced

¼ teaspoon sea salt

¼ teaspoon freshly ground black pepper

½ stalk celery, diced

2 tablespoons chives, diced

3 cups cooked salmon

BUNS

16 small bib lettuce leaves

In a medium bowl, mash the avocados with lemon juice. Mix in the salt, pepper, celery and chives. Flake the salmon into smaller-than-bite-size pieces and fold it into the mixture.

Wash and dry the lettuce and set aside.

Fill eight lettuce leaves evenly with the salmon salad and top each with the remaining lettuce.

PER SERVING: Calories: 520, Fat: 32g, Protein: 45g, Sodium: 780mg, Fiber: 13g, Carbohydrates: 19g, Sugar: 6g

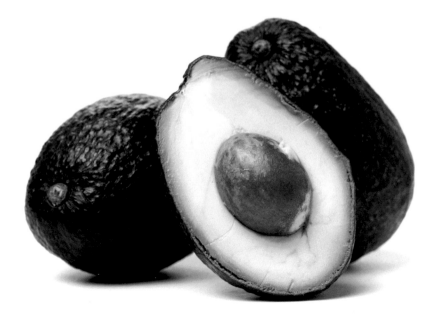

ASIAN SKILLET SALMON

A simple sauce makes this Asian-inspired salmon dish one that you'll come to rely on during busy weeknights.

INGREDIENTS **DIRECTIONS** **SERVES 4**

- 2 cloves garlic, chopped
- 2 tablespoons Pegan Ketchup (page 73)
- 1 teaspoon soy sauce
- 1 teaspoon mustard
- 2 teaspoons honey
- 2 dashes hot sauce
- 2 tablespoons olive oil
- 4 salmon fillets

Combine first six ingredients in a small saucepan over medium-low. Cook about 5 minutes, stirring frequently. The sauce will be thick. Remove it from heat. Spread half of the mixture evenly over each piece of salmon.

Rub oil on the bottom of the salmon and place on a hot cast-iron pan, skin-side down. Cover and cook about 10 minutes, depending on the size of the fillet. Place the salmon on a serving platter and brush with remaining sauce.

PER SERVING: Calories: 354, Fat: 21g, Protein: 35g, Sodium: 249mg, Fiber: 0g, Carbohydrates: 5.4g, Sugar: 4.7g

VEGETABLE AND MUSSELS BOWL

You can skip the mussels to make a simple soup, but we don't suggest that you do—the brine adds a delicious depth to the Vegetable Chop.

INGREDIENTS **DIRECTIONS** **SERVES 4**

- 2 pounds mussels
- 2 cups Vegetable Chop (page 146)
- 1 cup vegetable broth
- 2 tablespoons fresh parsley, chopped

Scrub the mussels with water and a sponge to clean off any debris. Pull the hairy ends off each mussel to debeard them.

Blend together 1 cup Vegetable Chop with the broth in a blender until smooth.

Add the blended mixture to a skillet with the remaining cup of Vegetable Chop. Warm the vegetables over medium heat and add the mussels, cover and cook until most of the mussels open, about 5 minutes. Discard any unopened mussels.

Divide the mussels among four bowls and top with parsley.

PER SERVING: Calories: 480, Fat: 16g, Protein: 57g, Sodium: 1,011mg, Fiber: 3.2g, Carbohydrates: 26g, Sugar: 2.6g

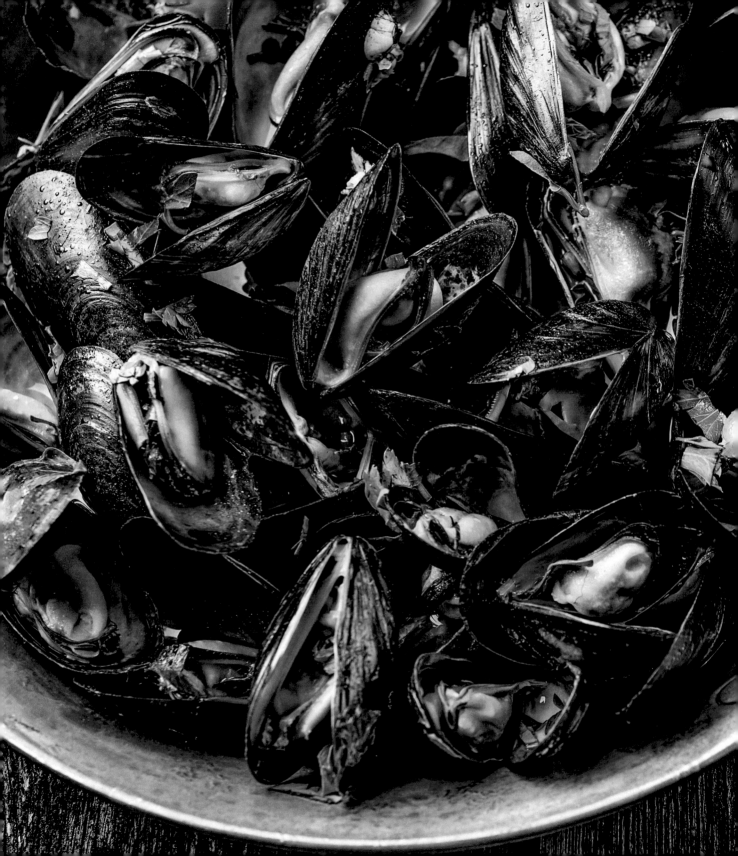

BUFFALO CAULIFLOWER LETTUCE CUPS

Butter lettuce leaves make for ideal "cups" that can be filled with anything you'd like—and this combination of spicy, crunchy and creamy ingredients is especially good.

INGREDIENTS

- 1 cup almond flour
- ¾ cup water
- ½ teaspoon garlic powder
- ½ teaspoon onion powder
- ½ teaspoon sea salt
- ½ teaspoon freshly ground black pepper
- 1 head cauliflower
- 2 tablespoons olive oil
- 1 cup hot sauce
- 8 large butter lettuce leaves
- 2 cups Apple Cucumber Coleslaw (page 132)
- 1 cup Avocado Crema (page 163)

DIRECTIONS

SERVES 4

Preheat oven to 375 degrees F.

In a medium bowl, mix together the flour, water, garlic powder, onion powder, salt and pepper.

Wash the cauliflower and cut it into florets. Line a cookie sheet with parchment paper and brush olive oil onto paper. Coat all of the florets with the batter and place them onto the cookie sheet.

Bake for 20 to 30 minutes, or until fork-tender, turning once during cooking.

Remove the cookie sheet from the oven and pour the hot sauce over the florets; coat all sides by gently turning with a spatula.

Take the lettuce leaves, evenly fill each with the buffalo cauliflower, top each with an even amount of coleslaw and drizzle with the Avocado Crema.

PER SERVING: Calories: 461, Fat: 34g, Protein: 14g, Sodium: 574mg, Fiber: 15g, Carbohydrates: 32g, Sugar: 12g

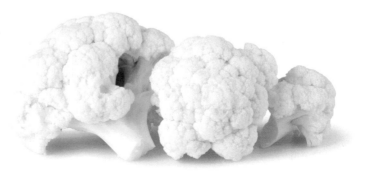

STUFFED POBLANO PEPPERS

These stuffed peppers are a great make-ahead meal—just stuff them ahead of time and pop them in the oven when you're ready.

INGREDIENTS

DIRECTIONS

SERVES 4

PEPPERS

4 poblano peppers

1 tablespoon olive oil

CHIPOTLE SAUCE

1 tablespoon tomato paste

1 tablespoon apple cider vinegar

1 teaspoon chipotle powder (or smoked paprika/cayenne powder mix)

½ teaspoon cumin

¼ teaspoon oregano

¼ teaspoon garlic powder

¼ teaspoon salt

FILLING

2 pounds boneless chicken breasts

4 cups prepared Cauliflower Fried Black Rice (page 136)

¼ cup cilantro

AVOCADO CREMA

2 ripe avocados

¼ cup chopped cilantro

1 lime, juiced

2 tablespoons avocado oil

¼ teaspoon sea salt

¼ teaspoon cumin

GARNISH

2 sliced avocados

Small bunch fresh cilantro

Lightly brush the whole poblano peppers with oil. Roast the peppers over the open flame of a gas stove or grill until charred and blistered.

Preheat oven to 400 degrees F.

Let the peppers cool until they are able to be handled, and peel away the skin. Cut a slit down one side to open the pepper and remove seeds. Set aside.

In a small bowl, mix together all chipotle sauce ingredients.

Cover the chicken with the sauce and place in a nonstick frying pan with oil. Cook over medium heat for 4 minutes on each side, or until internal temperature reaches 165 degrees F. Let the chicken cool enough to handle. Shred the chicken with two forks and mix with any remaining sauce.

Mix together the chicken, Cauliflower Fried Black Rice and cilantro in a medium bowl.

Evenly fill the peppers with filling. Place the peppers in a baking dish covered with foil. Place in the oven and cook for 25 to 30 minutes.

Meanwhile, place all crema ingredients in a blender and blend until smooth.

Remove the peppers from the oven, drizzle with the crema and garnish with avocado and cilantro.

PER SERVING: Calories: 893, Fat: 50g, Protein: 67g, Sodium: 1,336mg, Fiber: 25g, Carbohydrates: 54g, Sugar: 19g

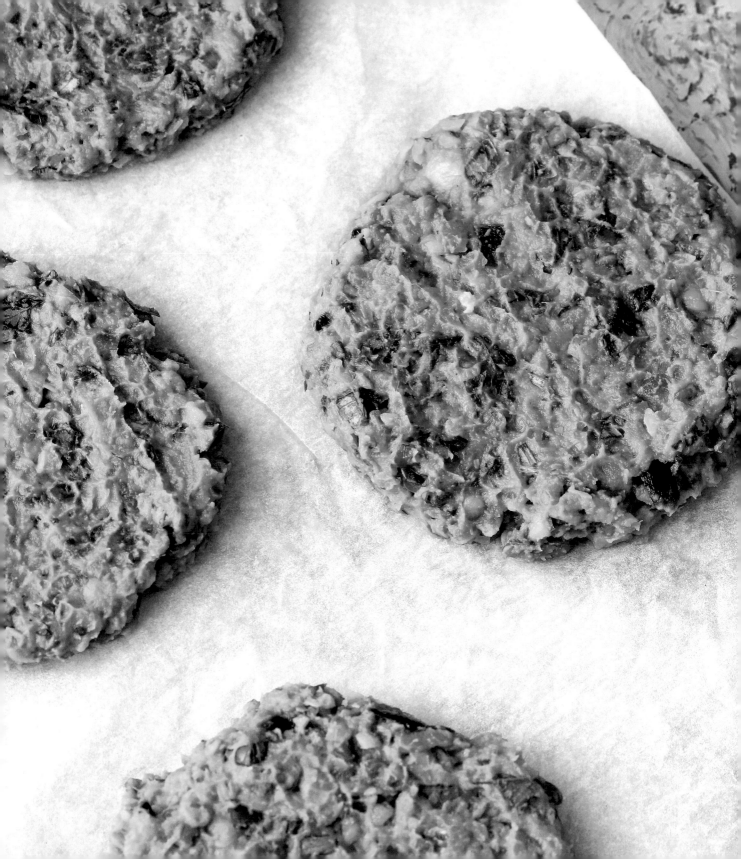

QUINOA AND SWEET POTATO BURGER

These tasty burgers are a good source of fiber and potassium. They can be made ahead of time—freeze them individually so you can grab a burger whenever you want.

| INGREDIENTS | DIRECTIONS | SERVES 4 |

INGREDIENTS

- 3 cups peeled, cubed sweet potatoes
- 3 tablespoons olive oil, divided
- ½ teaspoon sea salt
- ½ teaspoon freshly ground black pepper
- 1 cup leeks, chopped
- 2 cloves garlic, minced
- 3 eggs
- 1 teaspoon fresh rosemary, minced
- 1 teaspoon red pepper flakes
- 3 cups prepared quinoa
- 8 large butter lettuce leaves

DIRECTIONS

Preheat oven to 350 degrees F.

Place sweet potatoes on a parchment-lined cookie sheet with 1 tablespoon oil, salt and pepper. Mix to coat evenly. Cook for 20 minutes, or until fork-tender.

In a frying pan over medium-low heat, add 1 tablespoon oil and cook leeks and garlic until tender, about 3 to 4 minutes.

In a small bowl, mix together the eggs.

In a large bowl, add the sweet potatoes, cooked leeks and garlic and the remaining burger ingredients. Add the eggs and mix together, crushing the sweet potato slightly while mixing. Make four large patties.

In a large nonstick skillet over medium heat, add the remaining oil and cook the burgers on each side for about 4 minutes, or until cooked through. Place each burger on a lettuce leaf and top each with the remaining lettuce.

Optional: Serve with Garden Vegetable Spread (page 55) or Avocado Crema (page 163) or both, and top with Apple Cucumber Coleslaw (page 132).

PER SERVING: Calories: 691, Fat: 18g, Protein: 25g, Sodium: 561mg, Fiber: 13g, Carbohydrates: 107g, Sugar: 5.7g

ORANGE PEPPER PESTO-STUFFED ROASTED CABBAGE STEAKS

This healthy "steak" is served with a healthy and delicious pesto.
It's a recipe you'll reach for often, especially if you have vegan guests.

INGREDIENTS

ORANGE PEPPER PESTO

- 2 orange peppers
- ¼ cup pine nuts
- 2 cloves garlic
- ½ cup olive oil
- 1 tablespoon horseradish
- ½ teaspoon sea salt

CABBAGE STEAKS

- 1 large dark green cabbage
- 2 tablespoons olive oil
- ½ teaspoon sea salt
- ½ teaspoon freshly ground black pepper
- ¼ cup fresh parsley, chopped

DIRECTIONS

SERVES 4

Preheat oven to 375 degrees F.

Roast the peppers over the open flame of a gas stove or grill until charred and blistered. Let the peppers sit to cool and remove the skin, stem and seeds.

In a small saucepan, lightly toast the pine nuts over medium-low heat for about 3 minutes. Watch carefully, making sure they don't burn.

Place the roasted pepper, pine nuts and the remaining pesto ingredients in a food processor and blend until smooth.

Remove the outer leaves from the cabbage and trim the stalk. Slice the cabbage into ½-inch "steaks."

Line a cookie sheet with parchment paper and grease with 1 tablespoon oil. Place the cabbage steaks onto the cookie sheet and brush the remaining oil onto each cabbage steak and season with salt and pepper.

Spread pesto onto each steak and press into the cabbage.

Place in the preheated oven on the middle rack and cook for about 20 minutes, or until fork-tender. Cover with foil during cooking if they get too brown. Garnish with parsley and serve.

PER SERVING: Calories: 479, Fat: 40g, Protein: 6.2g, Sodium: 753mg, Fiber: 6.4g, Carbohydrates: 29g, Sugar: 11g

MUSHROOM STEW

Shiitake mushrooms have a surprisingly rich taste, plus they support heart health and immune function—they make for a pretty powerful mushroom stew!

INGREDIENTS	DIRECTIONS	SERVES 4

INGREDIENTS

- 2 tablespoons olive oil
- 1 pound shiitake mushrooms
- 1 shallot, diced
- 2 cloves garlic, minced
- 2 sprigs fresh thyme
- ¼ cup vegetable broth
- ¼ teaspoon sea salt
- ¼ teaspoon freshly ground black pepper
- 2 tablespoons fresh parsley, chopped

DIRECTIONS

In a medium skillet over medium-high heat, add oil and cook the mushrooms until starting to brown. Lower the heat to medium-low. Add the shallots, garlic, thyme, broth, salt and pepper.

Simmer the mushrooms until softened and the liquid has reduced by ¼. Discard the thyme sprigs. Garnish with parsley. Serve over Roasted and Mashed Turnips (page 145) or Roasted Garlic and Herb Millet Polenta (page 157) if desired.

PER SERVING: Calories: 116, Fat: 7.2g, Protein: 4.3g, Sodium: 16mg, Fiber: 4.5g, Carbohydrates: 11g, Sugar: 1.3g

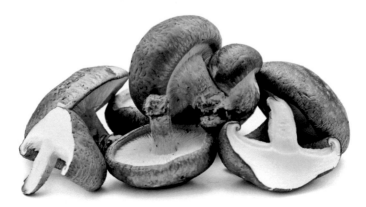

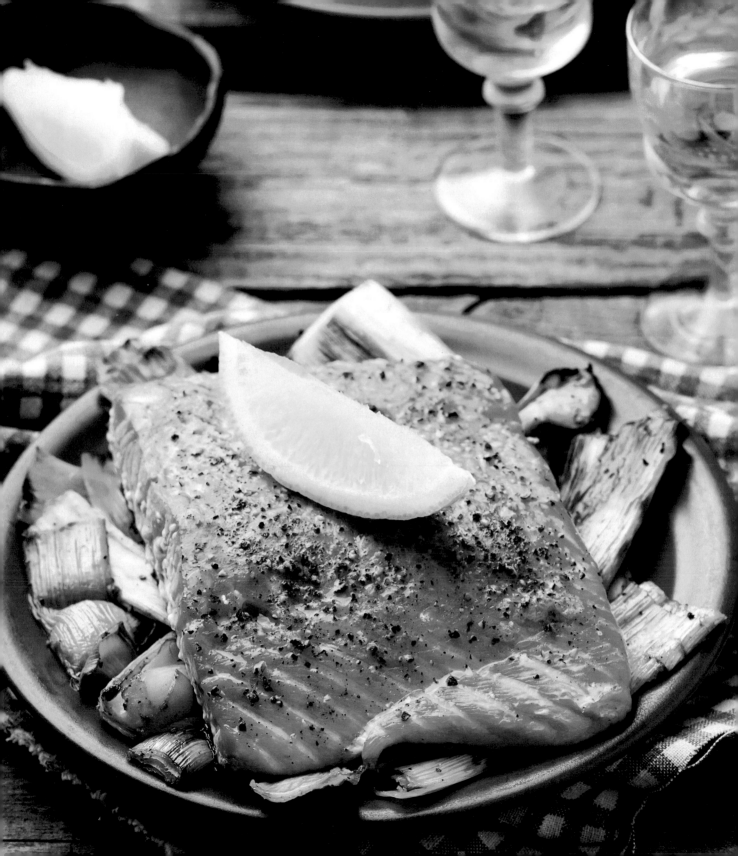

SKILLET BRAISED SALMON AND VEGETABLES

There's nothing like a good one-pot meal. A large, heavy-bottomed
Dutch oven is perfect for this braise.

INGREDIENTS

- 1 leek
- 1 red bell pepper
- 2 cloves garlic
- 1 head cauliflower
- 1 tablespoon olive oil
- ½ pound fresh spinach
- 2½ cups almond milk
- 2½ cups vegetable broth
- 4 salmon fillets
- ½ teaspoon sea salt
- ½ teaspoon freshly ground black pepper
- ¼ teaspoon freshly grated turmeric
- 4 tablespoons arrowroot
- ½ cup water
- 1 tablespoon fresh parsley, chopped

DIRECTIONS

Wash all vegetables. Cut the leeks in half lengthwise, keeping the root intact, and run under cold water to rinse out any sand. Cut off the root and slice the white and light-green part of the leeks.

Dice the red pepper, mince the garlic and cut the cauliflower into florets.

In a large skillet over medium heat, add the olive oil. Cook the leeks and red bell pepper for a couple of minutes, stir in the garlic and spinach and cook for another minute. Stir in the milk and broth and simmer to reduce sauce by ¼, about 5 minutes. Add in the salmon and cauliflower, seasoning with salt, pepper and turmeric. Cover and continue to cook for 10 to 12 minutes, or until salmon reaches an internal temperature of 140 degrees F.

In a small bowl, whisk together the water and arrowroot. Add it into the skillet and simmer a couple of minutes to thicken. Garnish with parsley.

Optional: Serve over Cauliflower Fried Black Rice (page 136).

PER SERVING: Calories: 448, Fat: 20g, Protein: 43g, Sodium: 567mg, Fiber: 8g, Carbohydrates: 29g, Sugar: 7.1g

SERVES 4

MEDITERRANEAN VEGETABLE SHRIMP SCAMPI

Shrimp scampi can sometimes be too rich—the addition of vegetables
in the Pegan version elevates both the nutrition and the taste!

INGREDIENTS

- 3 small zucchini
- 4 tablespoons olive oil
- 7 cloves garlic, minced
- ½ red pepper, diced
- 1 cup cremini mushrooms, chopped
- ½ red onion, diced
- 1 cup tomatoes, diced
- ¼ cup Kalamata olives, pitted, chopped
- 1 cup vegetable broth
- 1 tablespoon fresh basil, chopped
- 1 tablespoon fresh parsley, chopped
- 16 jumbo shrimp, peeled, deveined, with tails on

DIRECTIONS

SERVES 4

With a spiralizer or mandolin slicer fitted with a julienne attachment, slice the zucchini into noodles. Set aside.

In a large nonstick skillet over medium heat, add the oil. Cook the garlic, red pepper, mushrooms, onions, tomatoes and olives for 4 to 5 minutes, stirring often. Stir in the broth, basil and parsley and simmer for 3 minutes. Add the shrimp and zucchini to the skillet and cook until the shrimp is pink and no longer opaque.

Transfer to bowls and serve.

PER SERVING: Calories: 355, Fat: 20g, Protein: 32g, Sodium: 606mg, Fiber: 3.7g, Carbohydrates: 14g, Sugar: 7.1g

CHICKEN AND PINEAPPLE SKEWERS

Pineapples are good for you; they alleviate inflammation and improve joint health. However, they are also high in sugar, so make sure to share these skewers with a friend!

INGREDIENTS

SKEWERS

- 1 pound chicken, cut into bite-size pieces
- 3 cups pineapple chunks (1-inch pieces)
- 1 red onion, sliced into 1-inch slices
- 3 cups cherry tomatoes
- 3 tablespoons olive oil
- 2 garlic cloves, minced
- ½ teaspoon salt
- ½ teaspoon paprika
- ½ teaspoon pepper
- ½ teaspoon cayenne
- ½ teaspoon dried parsley
- Zest of ½ lime

GARNISH

- 4 green onions, diced
- Zest of ½ lime

DIRECTIONS

SERVES 4

Place the chicken, pineapple, red onion and tomatoes onto metal skewers or wooden skewers that have been soaked in water.

In a small bowl, mix together the oil, garlic, salt, paprika, pepper, cayenne, parsley and lime zest. Brush each skewer with the spice mixture.

On a hot grill, cook the skewers on all sides until the skewers are lightly charred and the chicken has reached an internal temperature of 165 degrees F, about 2 to 3 minutes on each side.

Garnish with the green onion and lime zest.

PER SERVING: Calories: 305, Fat: 11g, Protein: 28g, Sodium: 539mg, Fiber: 3.7g, Carbohydrates: 26g, Sugar: 17g

SLOW COOKER PULLED PORK

Serve this simple slow-cooker meal over Roasted and Mashed Turnips (page 145) or topped with Apple Cucumber Coleslaw (page 132).

INGREDIENTS   **DIRECTIONS**   SERVES 4

1 onion, diced

3 cloves garlic, minced

1 cup chicken broth

1 teaspoon sea salt

1 teaspoon freshly ground black pepper

2 pounds pork butt

2 cups Pegan Ketchup (page 73)

¼ cup honey

1 tablespoon chili powder

Place the onions, garlic and broth on the bottom of the slow cooker. Season the pork with salt and pepper and place the pork on top of the onions. Cook for 6 to 8 hours on high or 8 to 10 hours on low.

Take the meat from the slow cooker and place it on a cutting board. Remove any fat and bone from the meat. Shred the meat with two forks, pulling apart into bite-size pieces. Remove all but ½ cup liquid from the slow cooker and stir in the Pegan Ketchup, honey and chili powder. Serve the pulled pork with as much sauce as you like.

PER SERVING: Calories: 906, Fat: 49g, Protein: 53g, Sodium: 1,831mg, Fiber: 0.9g, Carbohydrates: 54g, Sugar: 50g

STUFFED MEATLOAF

Stuffing this meatloaf with roasted vegetables adds a much-needed nutritional boost to classic comfort food.

INGREDIENTS   **DIRECTIONS**   SERVES 4

¾ pound 80/20 ground beef

2 cups Vegetable Chop (page 146)

2 cups fresh baby spinach

1 cup Pegan Ketchup (page 73)

Preheat oven to 375 degrees F.

Cut a piece of parchment paper in a large square, about 14-by-14 inches. Place the beef on the parchment and flatten out to a 12-by-12-inch square. Evenly spread 1 cup Vegetable Chop on the meat, then top with half of the baby spinach, then the remaining Vegetable Chop and remaining spinach. Roll as you would a jelly roll and place seam-side down into an oven-safe baking dish. Top with the Pegan Ketchup and place in the preheated oven.

Cook on the middle rack for 30 to 40 minutes, or until the meat is cooked through.

PER SERVING: Calories: 384, Fat: 19g, Protein: 26g, Sodium: 820mg, Fiber: 3.6g, Carbohydrates: 26g, Sugar: 18g

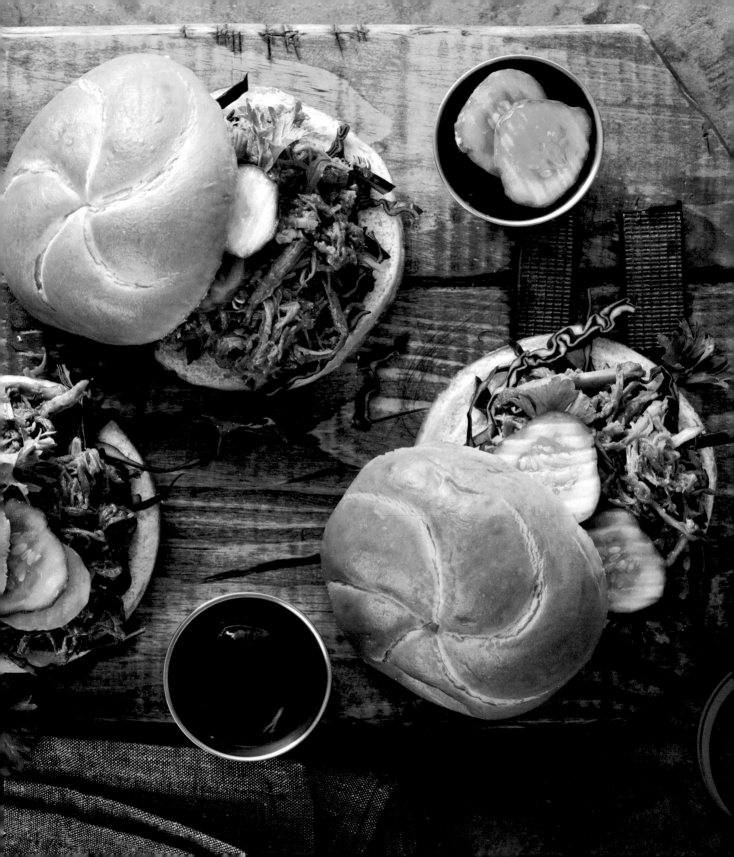

SEARED SCALLOPS OVER GREEN BEANS, TOMATOES AND MICROGREENS

Fresh ingredients shine in this colorful and good-for-you dish—you'll be looking forward to dinner all day.

INGREDIENTS

BEANS AND TOMATOES

- 1 tablespoon olive oil
- 1 pound green beans
- 1 pint grape tomatoes
- ¼ teaspoon salt
- ¼ teaspoon freshly ground black pepper
- 2 cloves garlic, minced
- 1 tablespoon parsley, chopped

SCALLOPS

- 1 tablespoon ghee
- 1 pound scallops
- 2 cloves garlic, minced
- ½ teaspoon sea salt
- ¼ teaspoon freshly ground black pepper

MICROGREENS

- 1½ cups microgreens
- ½ lemon, juice and zest
- 1 anchovy, finely chopped
- ¼ cup olive oil
- ¼ teaspoon red pepper flakes
- ¼ teaspoon sea salt

DIRECTIONS

SERVES 4

In a large skillet over medium heat, add the oil and green beans. Cook the beans about 10 minutes, stirring often. Add the tomatoes, salt and pepper. Continue to cook until the beans and tomatoes are just tender, about 4 more minutes. Add the garlic and parsley and cook another minute.

In a medium nonstick pan over medium-high heat, add the ghee and garlic and sear the scallops for a couple of minutes on each side, or until scallops are no longer opaque. Add salt and pepper.

Wash the microgreens. In a container or jar with a top, add all dressing ingredients and shake to combine. Toss the microgreens with the dressing.

Transfer the green bean–and-tomato mixture to a serving dish. Top with the seared scallops and dressed microgreens.

PER SERVING: Calories: 347, Fat: 22g, Protein: 19g, Sodium: 984mg, Fiber: 6.5g, Carbohydrates: 20g, Sugar: 2.9g

SLOW COOKER CHICKEN CACCIATORE

There's nothing better than coming home to a hot meal that smells delicious. Don't count on having any leftovers!

INGREDIENTS

- 2 tablespoons olive oil
- 8 bone-in chicken thighs
- 1 cup chicken broth, divided
- 1 (28-ounce) can crushed tomatoes
- ½ green pepper, diced
- 1 onion, diced
- 3 cloves garlic, minced
- 7 large fresh basil leaves, chopped
- ½ teaspoon fresh thyme leaves
- ¼ teaspoon fresh rosemary, chopped fine

DIRECTIONS

In a large nonstick skillet over medium heat, add oil and fry the chicken on both sides until the skin is browned. Fry in batches to avoid crowding the pan.

Pour out the oil from the pan and discard. Add ½ cup broth to deglaze the pan, scraping up any browned bits. Place the chicken and pan juices into the slow cooker, then add all other ingredients.

Cover and cook on high for 3 to 4 hours or on low for 4 to 6 hours.

SERVES 4

PER SERVING: Calories: 361, Fat: 21g, Protein: 26g, Sodium: 207mg, Fiber: 3.8g, Carbohydrates: 19g, Sugar: 11g

STUFFED EGGPLANT

Chia seeds add extra fiber and nutrients to this classic Italian dish.

INGREDIENTS

2 small eggplants

2 tablespoons salt, plus 1 teaspoon

Drizzle olive oil

½ pound ground beef

1 onion, diced

2 cups tomatoes, chopped

2 tablespoons chia seeds

4 cloves garlic, diced

1 tablespoon chopped fresh basil

1 teaspoon chopped fresh parsley

1 teaspoon freshly ground black pepper

2 eggs

1 cup marinara sauce, homemade or store-bought

DIRECTIONS

SERVES 4

Preheat oven to 350 degrees F.

Cut the eggplants in half lengthwise. Scoop out the flesh leaving ¼ inch around the edges. Cut the scooped eggplant into small ½-inch pieces.

Salt the eggplant cubes with 2 tablespoons salt. Place in a mesh strainer in the sink or over a bowl to catch the bitter liquid. Let sit for 30 minutes.

Rinse salt off the eggplants and place in a large skillet with olive oil, beef, onions, tomatoes, chia seeds, garlic, basil, parsley, pepper and remaining salt. Cook over medium heat for about 7 minutes, stirring often. Let mixture cool.

In a small bowl, mix eggs, then add to the skillet and mix stuffing thoroughly.

Evenly stuff each eggplant. Top each eggplant with marinara sauce.

Bake the stuffed eggplants for 45 minutes.

PER SERVING: Calories: 404, Fat: 23g, Protein: 24g, Sodium: 3,631mg, Fiber: 12g, Carbohydrates: 30g, Sugar: 15g

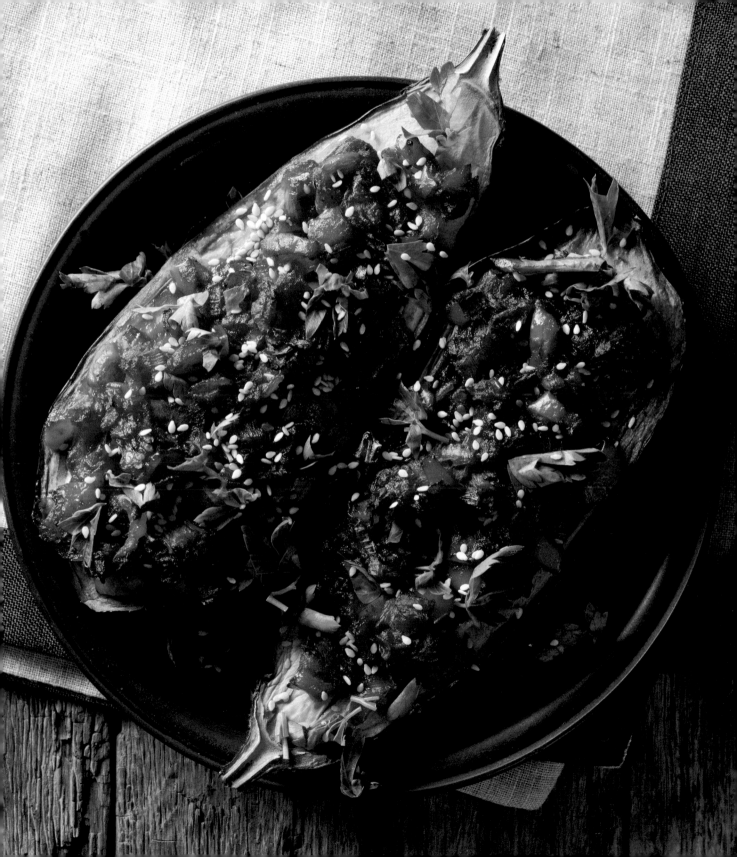

SHRIMP DINNER POCKETS

As the pockets cook, the flavors meld together and the shrimp juices and seasoning slowly flavor the vegetables. Serve these right in the foil—it's like getting a little present.

INGREDIENTS

1 pound jumbo shrimp

2 tablespoons blackened seasoning

1 pound purple fingerling potatoes, sliced in half

2 medium zucchinis, sliced

1 shallot, sliced

2 cups cremini mushrooms, wiped clean, sliced

8 green onions, washed

4 tablespoons olive oil

1 tablespoon sea salt

1 tablespoon freshly ground black pepper

DIRECTIONS

SERVES 4

Preheat grill to medium-high heat (about 425 degrees F).

Peel and devein the shrimp. Add the shrimp to a bowl and toss with blackened seasoning.

Wash the potatoes and prick with a fork. Place in a microwave-safe bowl and cook for 3 to 4 minutes, or until the potatoes are softened.

In four large double-lined foil sheets, evenly add the potatoes, zucchini, shallots, creminis and whole green onion. Place a tablespoon of oil on top of the vegetables and season with salt and pepper. Pull the foil sides up to create a pouch. Place the shrimp on top and wrap the foil tightly closed. Place on the hot grill and cook for 10 to 12 minutes. Remove from the grill and carefully open the pouch—they will be steamy.

PER SERVING: Calories: 391, Fat: 16g, Protein: 35g, Sodium: 793mg, Fiber: 3.7g, Carbohydrates: 28g, Sugar: 7.3g

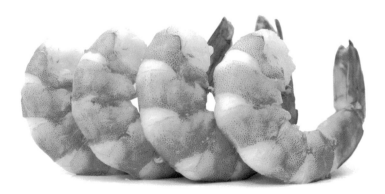

SOBA NOODLES AND CLAM SAUCE

Soba is an excellent substitution for regular pastas and a delicious bed for these small, sweet littleneck clams and garlicky sauce.

INGREDIENTS

- 2 pounds littleneck clams
- 12 ounces soba noodles
- ½ cup chicken or vegetable broth
- 3 cloves garlic, minced
- 1 green onion, chopped
- 1 lemon, juice and zest
- 2 tablespoons fresh parsley, chopped

DIRECTIONS

SERVES 4

Place the clams in a large bowl covered with water (this cleans the clams as the clams will spit out the sand). Discard the sandy water and add fresh water, repeating until the water stays clean and no more sand is visible, about 20 minutes.

Boil a large pot of water and add the soba noodles. Boil for about 4 to 5 minutes, or until al dente. Drain the noodles and return to the pot, off the heat.

In a large skillet, add the broth, garlic, onion and lemon. Bring to a simmer over medium heat. Cook the broth until reduced by ¼. Add in the clams and cover for 5 to 10 minutes, or until most of the clams are wide-open. Discard any clams that do not open.

Add the noodles to a large bowl, top with the clams and sprinkle with parsley.

PER SERVING: Calories: 361, Fat: 4.2g, Protein: 63g, Sodium: 319mg, Fiber: 0.1g, Carbohydrates: 20g, Sugar: 0.6g

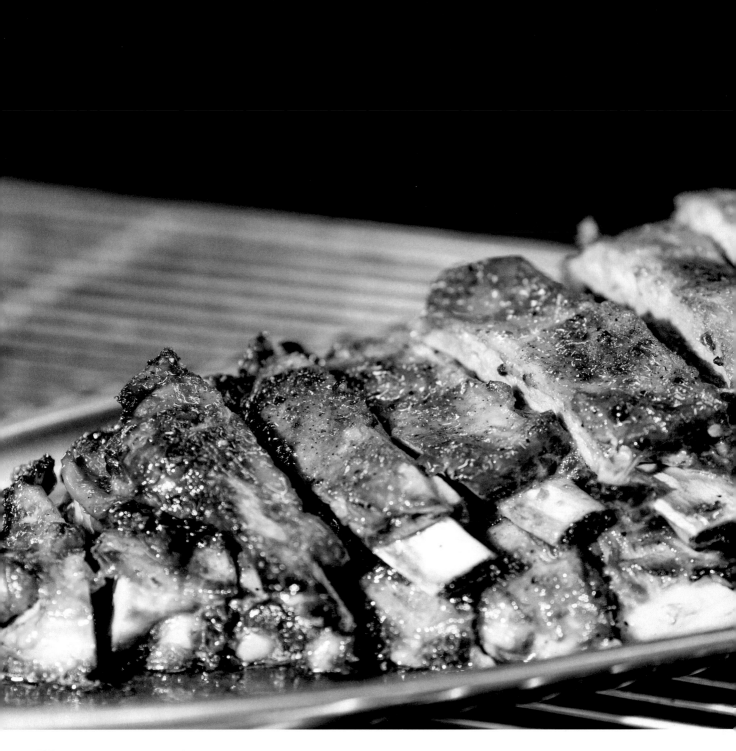

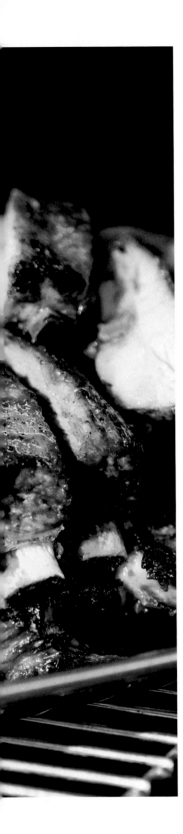

THAI ORANGE GINGER BABY BACK RIBS

This orange ginger sauce takes baby back ribs to a whole new level! You may want to make extra—these will go fast.

INGREDIENTS

RIBS

- 1 rack baby back ribs
- ½ teaspoon sea salt
- ½ teaspoon freshly ground black pepper

ORANGE GINGER SAUCE

- Zest and juice of 1 orange
- 1 tablespoon fresh ginger
- 2 cloves garlic, minced
- ¼ teaspoon red pepper flakes
- 2 tablespoons soy sauce
- 2 tablespoons tahini

DIRECTIONS   SERVES 2-4

Preheat oven to 325 degrees F.

Remove the silver skin from under the ribs, season with salt and pepper and wrap the ribs in foil. Place the wrapped ribs on a sheet pan and place them in the oven to cook 3½ hours.

Combine all orange ginger sauce ingredients in a blender and blend until smooth. Set aside.

Take the ribs out of the oven and drain off the fat. Using half of the orange ginger sauce, brush the top of the ribs with sauce. Set the oven to broil, place the ribs back into the oven to caramelize the sauce—this should take about 3 minutes, but watch carefully so the sauce does not burn.

Remove from the oven and serve with any extra sauce.

PER SERVING: Calories: 341, Fat: 25g, Protein: 23g, Sodium: 1,002mg, Fiber: 1.6g, Carbohydrates: 7.3g, Sugar: 3.2g

ARTISAN TOMATO SANDWICH WITH HEALTHY SANDWICH SPREAD

Sometimes all you want and need is a simple tomato sandwich.
Wrapping garden-fresh tomatoes in lettuce makes for a fresh, tasty meal.

INGREDIENTS

HEALTHY SANDWICH SPREAD

- 2 avocados
- ⅔ cup ground pistachios
- ¼ teaspoon pepper
- ½ teaspoon ginger
- ¼ teaspoon turmeric
- ¼ teaspoon cayenne powder

SANDWICH

- 8 large romaine lettuce leaves
- 8–16 slices heirloom tomatoes (depends on size of tomato)
- 12 sprigs pea shoots
- 6 basil leaves
- ¼ teaspoon pepper
- 3 ounces artisan lettuce mix

DIRECTIONS

SERVES 4-6

With a blender, blend together all sandwich spread ingredients until smooth.

Place four romaine leaves onto a work surface. Top each piece of lettuce with a generous amount of the sandwich spread and an even amount of tomatoes, pea shoots, basil, pepper and lettuce mix. Spread a generous amount of sandwich spread onto the four remaining lettuce leaves. Place one on top of each sandwich, spread-side down.

Makes four sandwiches.

PER SERVING: Calories: 283, Fat: 21g, Protein: 9.4g, Sodium: 22mg, Fiber: 13g, Carbohydrates: 22g, Sugar: 7.7g

BEEF AND BROCCOLI

Skip the takeout and make this Chinese favorite at home.
Not only is it delicious, it's also faster than delivery.

INGREDIENTS	DIRECTIONS	SERVES 4-6

INGREDIENTS

- 2 heads broccoli
- 1 pound skirt steak
- ½ teaspoon sea salt
- ½ teaspoon freshly ground black pepper
- 1 teaspoon olive oil
- 2 cloves garlic, minced
- 1 teaspoon freshly grated ginger
- ⅓ cup soy sauce
- ¼ cup sesame oil
- 3 tablespoons honey
- 2 tablespoons sesame seeds

DIRECTIONS

Cut the broccoli into florets. Add the broccoli to a steamer basket fitted in a large pot of boiling water. Steam for about 10 minutes, or until the broccoli is just fork-tender.

Preheat the grill to medium-high.

Season the steak with salt and pepper. Cook the steaks 3 to 4 minutes on each side, or until medium-rare, with an internal temperature of 130 to 135 degrees F.

In a small saucepan coated with olive oil, cook the garlic and ginger for 1 minute. Remove from heat.

In a small bowl, mix together the soy sauce, garlic, ginger, sesame oil and honey.

Wipe out the small pan and toast the sesame seeds lightly over medium-low heat. Remove from the pan and set aside.

Cut the steak in half, then cut into thin slices against the grain of the meat.

Place the meat, broccoli, garlic mixture and sesame seeds onto a serving dish, stir to coat all ingredients and serve.

PER SERVING: Calories: 512, Fat: 28g, Protein: 34g, Sodium: 1,948mg, Fiber: 8.6g, Carbohydrates: 36g, Sugar: 18g

SWEDISH MEATBALLS

The mixture of beef and mushrooms makes these meatballs extra hearty.
If you'd like, make mini meatballs and serve them on toothpicks as an appetizer.

INGREDIENTS

MEATBALLS

- 2 tablespoons olive oil, divided
- 1 cup cremini mushrooms, finely chopped
- 2 cloves garlic, minced
- 1½ pounds ground beef
- 1 tablespoon dried basil
- 1 tablespoon dried parsley
- ½ teaspoon salt
- ½ teaspoon freshly ground black pepper
- ¼ cup water
- 2 eggs

SAUCE

- ½ cup chicken broth
- 1 tablespoon mustard
- ¼ cup sheep's yogurt
- ¼ teaspoon freshly ground black pepper

DIRECTIONS

SERVES 4

Preheat oven to 350 degrees F.

In a small frying pan over medium heat, add 1 tablespoon oil and cook the mushrooms until softened, about 3 minutes. Add the garlic and cook another minute. Let cool.

In a large bowl, mix the ground beef, cooled mushrooms and garlic, basil, parsley, salt, pepper and water.

In a small bowl, mix together the eggs. Add the eggs to the other ingredients.

Mix the ingredients together with your hands just until they are mixed well—do not overmix. Make golf ball–sized meatballs. Place on a parchment-lined sheet pan with remaining oil. Bake 10 to 15 minutes, or until the meatballs are cooked through.

In the same pan you cooked the mushrooms, add the sauce ingredients and simmer over medium-low heat until the sauce thickens slightly.

Place the meatballs on a serving dish, pour sauce on top and serve.

PER SERVING: Calories: 541, Fat: 33g, Protein: 51g, Sodium: 678mg, Fiber: 0g, Carbohydrates: 5.9g, Sugar: 2g

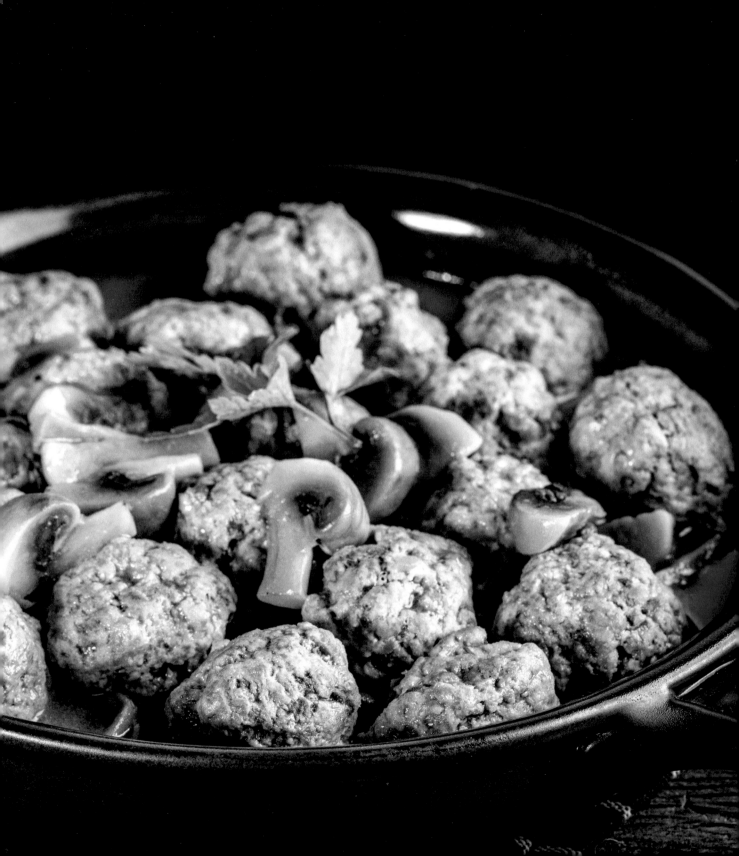

GRILLED PORK TENDERLOIN CHOPS WITH PLUM SAUCE

The trick to tender pork is to not overcook. A meat thermometer cuts out all the guesswork, guaranteeing juicy meat every time.

INGREDIENTS

PORK

- 2 pounds pork tenderloin
- 1 teaspoon salt
- 1 teaspoon pepper

SAUCE

- 4 plums, diced
- 3 tablespoons honey
- ½ teaspoon dried rosemary
- ½ teaspoon thyme
- 1 clove garlic, minced
- ½ teaspoon salt
- ⅓ cup water

DIRECTIONS

SERVES 6

Use cooking twine to tie the tenderloin together, using four ties at 1-inch intervals. Cut the pork into chops, leaving the twine tied in the middle of each chop. Season the chops with the salt and pepper. On a well-greased, hot grill, cook the chops on each side for about 4 minutes, or until cooked through. The internal temperature should be 145 degrees F.

Set the plums in a saucepan over medium-low heat with the honey, rosemary, thyme, garlic, salt and water. Cook sauce for about 10 minutes, or until the plums are soft and the sauce is thickened.

Take the pork tenderloin chops off the grill and let rest for 7 minutes. Place on a serving platter, drizzle with desired amount of sauce and serve.

PER SERVING: Calories: 439, Fat: 32g, Protein: 23g, Sodium: 600mg, Fiber: 0.7g, Carbohydrates: 14g, Sugar: 12g

SWEET POTATO BLACK BEAN CHILI

Sweet potatoes and black beans are always delicious together, but this chili is especially warming on a cold winter evening.

INGREDIENTS

- 3 tablespoons olive oil
- 1 large sweet onion, diced
- ½ red pepper, diced
- 3 cloves garlic, diced
- ¼ teaspoon fresh thyme, minced
- ¼ teaspoon fresh rosemary, minced
- 3 tablespoons chili powder
- 1 teaspoon cumin
- ¼ teaspoon salt
- ½ teaspoon freshly ground black pepper
- 2 (12.5-ounce) cans black beans, drained
- 3 cups vegetable broth
- 35 ounces canned Italian plum tomatoes, chopped
- 4 large sweet potatoes, peeled and chopped

DIRECTIONS

SERVES 4

In a large heavy-bottomed pot over medium-low heat, add the oil and cook the onions, peppers and garlic until vegetables start to soften but are not browned, about 3 to 4 minutes.

Stir in the herbs and spices, salt and pepper, and cook for another minute. Add in the remaining ingredients except potatoes and simmer for about 20 to 30 minutes to meld flavors and soften the beans. Place the potatoes into the chili and cook until the potatoes are tender, about 10 to 12 additional minutes.

Place a desired amount of chili into bowls and top with any of your favorite toppings, if desired.

PER SERVING: Calories: 543, Fat: 12g, Protein: 22g, Sodium: 847mg, Fiber: 23g, Carbohydrates: 87g, Sugar: 18g

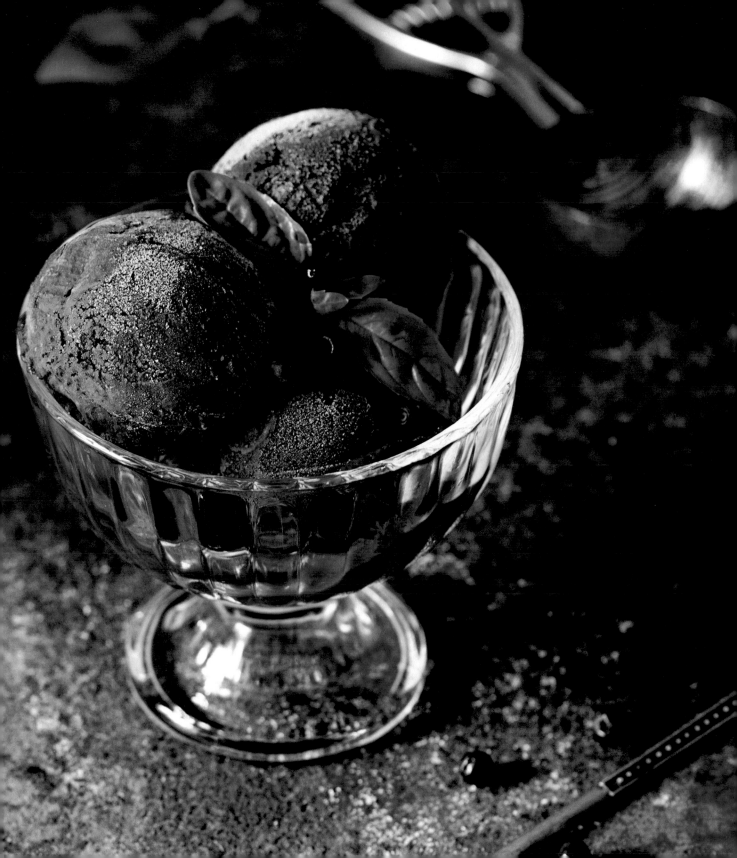

dessert

SAVE ROOM FOR SOMETHING SWEET.

Berry Cobbler 191

Raspberry Bars 192

Classic Baked Apples 193

Blood Orange Poached Pears 194

Black Rice Pudding with Dragon Fruit 197

Peppery Pudding 197

Blueberry Basil Ice Cream 199

Papaya Sherbet 199

Chocolate Bark 200

Chocolate Chip Skillet Brownies 202

Pudding-Filled Crepe Cake with Berries 205

Strawberry Cheesecake 206

Lemon Meringue Pie 209

Coconut, Matcha and Kiwi Parfait 210

Peanut Butter Cups 213

Meringue Cookies 214

Grilled Nectarines 217

Pumpkin Pie Parfait 218

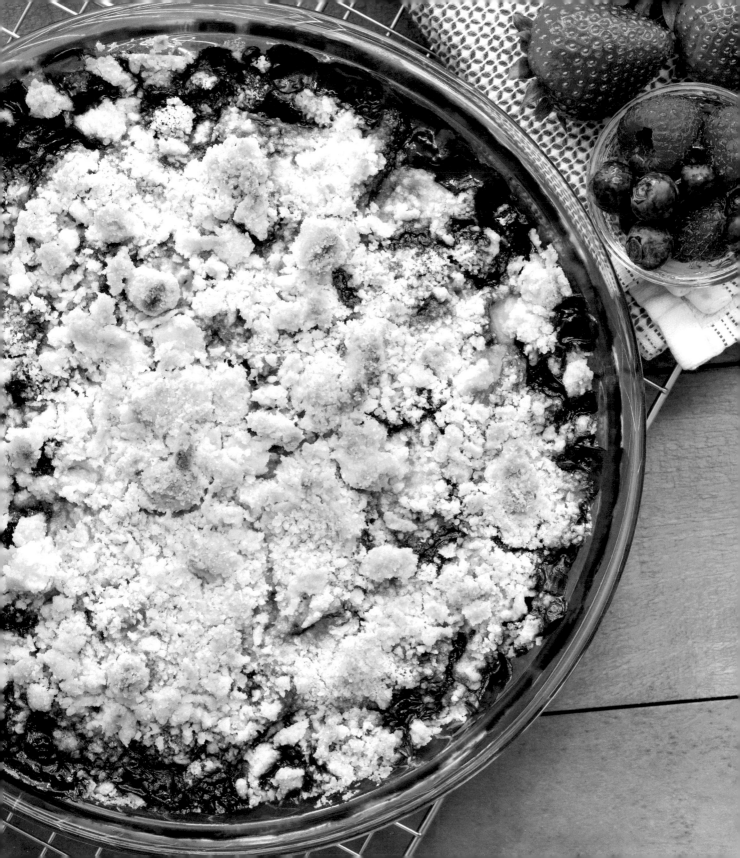

BERRY COBBLER

Bursting with color (and antioxidants!) from all the berries,
this cobbler is sure to be a hit at any gathering.

INGREDIENTS

FILLING

1 cup blueberries

1 cup blackberries

1 cup raspberries

1 cup strawberries

1 tablespoon coconut sugar

3 tablespoons fresh lemon juice

TOPPING

3 cups almond flour

½ cup pecans, chopped

¼ cup honey

1 teaspoon cinnamon

1 teaspoon vanilla

1 tablespoon butter, softened

DIRECTIONS

SERVES 8

Preheat oven to 375 degrees F.

Mix all filling ingredients together and place in the bottom of a greased 8-by-8-inch baking dish.

In a medium bowl, mix all topping ingredients together. Evenly cover the fruit with the topping.

Place in a preheated oven and bake for about 30 minutes, or until the fruit is bubbling and the topping is lightly browned. Let cool about 10 minutes before serving.

PER SERVING: Calories: 370, Fat: 28g, Protein: 10g, Sodium: 0.8mg, Fiber: 8.1g, Carbohydrates: 28g, Sugar: 16g

RASPBERRY BARS

These easy raspberry bars are a wonderful summer treat, but you can make them any time of year! Bring them to your next gathering and they'll soon become requested year round.

INGREDIENTS

DIRECTIONS

FILLING

  2 **cups fresh raspberries**

  ½ **teaspoon lemon juice**

  ½ **teaspoon honey**

  ¼ **teaspoon vanilla bean caviar**

  ¼ **cup water**

CRUST

  ⅔ **cup quinoa flakes, plus more for garnish**

  ⅔ **cup chopped walnuts**

  ½ **cup almond flour**

  ¼ **cup coconut sugar**

  ¼ **cup honey**

  ¼ **cup ground flaxseed**

  1 **teaspoon cinnamon**

  ¼ **teaspoon sea salt**

  2 **tablespoons coconut oil, more for greasing**

  1½ **tablespoons water**

Preheat oven to 350 degrees F.

In a medium saucepan over medium-low heat, add all filling ingredients and cook, stirring often, until the raspberries are soft and the mixture is thickened, about 10 minutes.

Add all crust ingredients together in a food processor and pulse until you reach a small gravel consistency.

Line an 8-by-8-inch baking dish with parchment paper. Grease the parchment paper with coconut oil. Take ¾ of the crust mixture and push it into the bottom of the baking dish. Bake the crust for 20 minutes.

Fill the crust with the raspberry mixture, and sprinkle the reserved crust mixture on top. Place back in the oven and cook for an additional 20 minutes.

Let cool and cut into 16 squares.

PER SERVING: Calories: 127, Fat: 7.5g, Protein: 2.6g, Sodium: 29mg, Fiber: 2.3g, Carbohydrates: 14g, Sugar: 8.9g

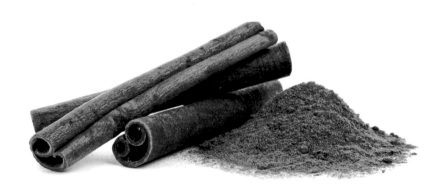

CLASSIC BAKED APPLES

When those crisp fall days come, there's nothing better to warm up with than baked apples. Plus, who doesn't love it when their kitchen smells like cinnamon, honey and almonds?

INGREDIENTS

DIRECTIONS

BAKED APPLES

4 large baking apples, such as honeycrisp

1½ cups almonds, crushed

2 tablespoons cinnamon

⅓ cup honey

½ lemon, juiced

Pinch salt

¼ cup water

WHIPPED CREAM (OPTIONAL)

1 can coconut cream, chilled overnight

⅛ teaspoon cream of tartar

2 tablespoons coconut sugar

Preheat oven to 350 degrees F.

Core the apples with an apple corer, leaving the bottoms intact. Take a paring knife and clean out any remaining core or seeds.

In a medium bowl, mix together the almonds, cinnamon, honey, lemon juice and salt.

Evenly place the mixture into each cored apple and set in an oven-safe baking dish. Add ¼ cup water to the bottom of the baking dish. Place in the preheated oven and bake about 45 minutes, or until the apples are soft.

Then, if you'd like, prepare the whipped cream. After chilling your coconut cream, half of the can will be a thick coconut milk and the other half will be a thick layer of coconut cream. Transfer the hard cream to the bowl of a stand mixer and reserve the liquid milk for another use.

Using the whisk attachment, beat the coconut cream with the cream of tartar in a stand mixer on medium. When the coconut cream begins to whip up and become light and fluffy, turn the mixer to high and slowly add in the sugar. Continue to beat until silky and hard peaks form.

Top the baked apples with whipped cream and serve.

PER SERVING: Calories: 336, Fat: 22g, Protein: 6.5g, Sodium: 79mg, Fiber: 6g, Carbohydrates: 33.5g, Sugar: 24g

BLOOD ORANGE POACHED PEARS

This elegant dessert could not be simpler to prepare, making it perfect for a dinner party or any night you want to treat yourself.

INGREDIENTS

- 4 Bosc pears, peeled
- 6 blood oranges, zest and juice
- 2 cups water
- 1 cup honey
- 1 teaspoon vanilla bean caviar
- 1 cinnamon stick
- Pinch salt

DIRECTIONS

SERVES 8

Place all ingredients in a Dutch oven, ensuring the pears are standing upright and submerged in liquid—add more water if necessary. Bring to a boil over medium-high. Reduce the heat to medium-low. Cover and simmer 1 hour, or until the pears are tender. Remove the pears from the pan using a slotted spoon.

PER SERVING: Calories: 183, Fat: 0.1g, Protein: 1g, Sodium: 76.5mg, Fiber: 4.6g, Carbohydrates: 48.5g, Sugar: 39.5g

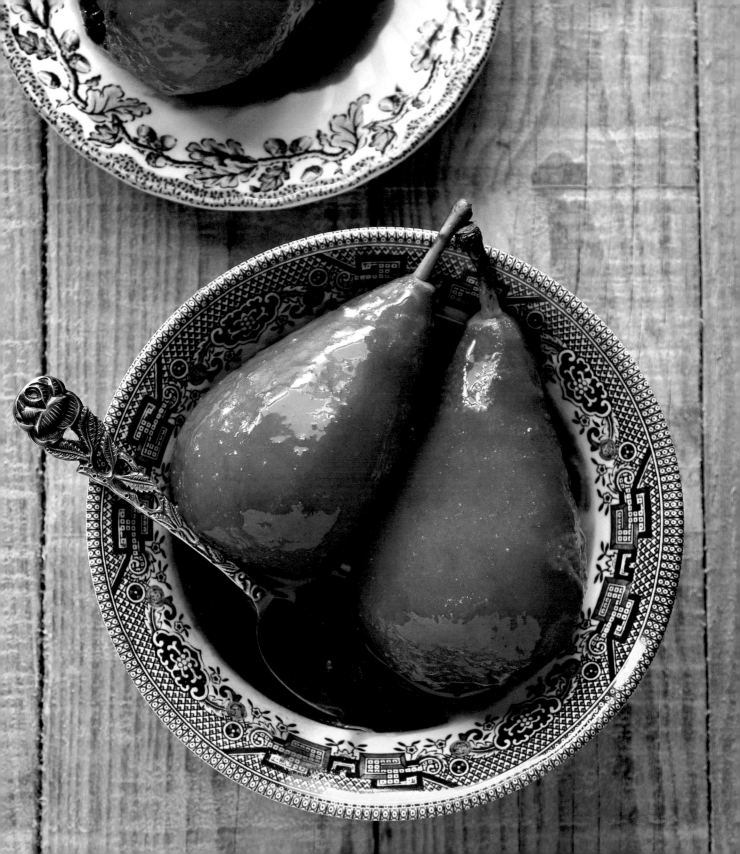

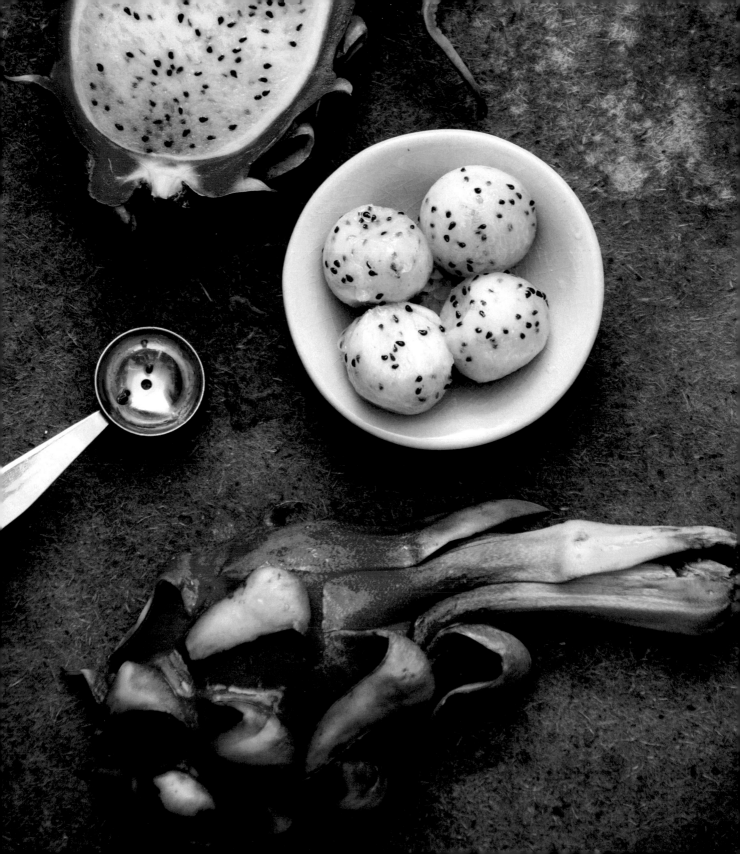

BLACK RICE PUDDING WITH DRAGON FRUIT

Black rice and dragon fruit add a dramatic touch to this delicious dessert!
But don't worry—it still tastes just like mom's homemade rice pudding.

INGREDIENTS

- ½ cup black rice
- 2 cups water
- 1 tablespoon cinnamon
- ¼ teaspoon vanilla bean caviar
- 1 cup unsweetened coconut milk
- ¼ cup coconut sugar
- ⅛ teaspoon sea salt
- 2 dragon fruits

DIRECTIONS   SERVES 4

In a heavy-bottomed saucepan, add rice and water. Cover and let simmer for 45 minutes, or until the rice is tender and the water has been absorbed. Mix in the cinnamon, vanilla, coconut milk, sugar and salt. Continue to cook until the mixture has thickened. Let cool to room temperature.

With a small melon baller, make balls from the dragon fruit. Place the rice pudding into serving dishes, leaving an inch on top. Top evenly with the dragon fruit balls and serve.

PER SERVING: Calories: 193, Fat: 10g, Protein: 2.6g, Sodium: 138mg, Fiber: 1.7g, Carbohydrates: 24g, Sugar: 17g

PEPPERY PUDDING

You can whip up this luscious treat in just a couple of minutes!
The sweet and the heat play off each other for a fun and tasty dessert.

INGREDIENTS

- 4 ripe avocados
- 4 tablespoons coconut sugar
- ¾ cup cocoa powder
- ¼ teaspoon vanilla bean caviar
- ½ teaspoon instant coffee
- ⅛ teaspoon salt
- 4 pinches crushed pink peppercorns

DIRECTIONS   SERVES 4

Place all ingredients except the pepper into a blender and blend until smooth. Place in four serving cups and sprinkle each with the pepper.

PER SERVING: Calories: 450, Fat: 33g, Protein: 10g, Sodium: 95mg, Fiber: 22g, Carbohydrates: 46g, Sugar: 20g

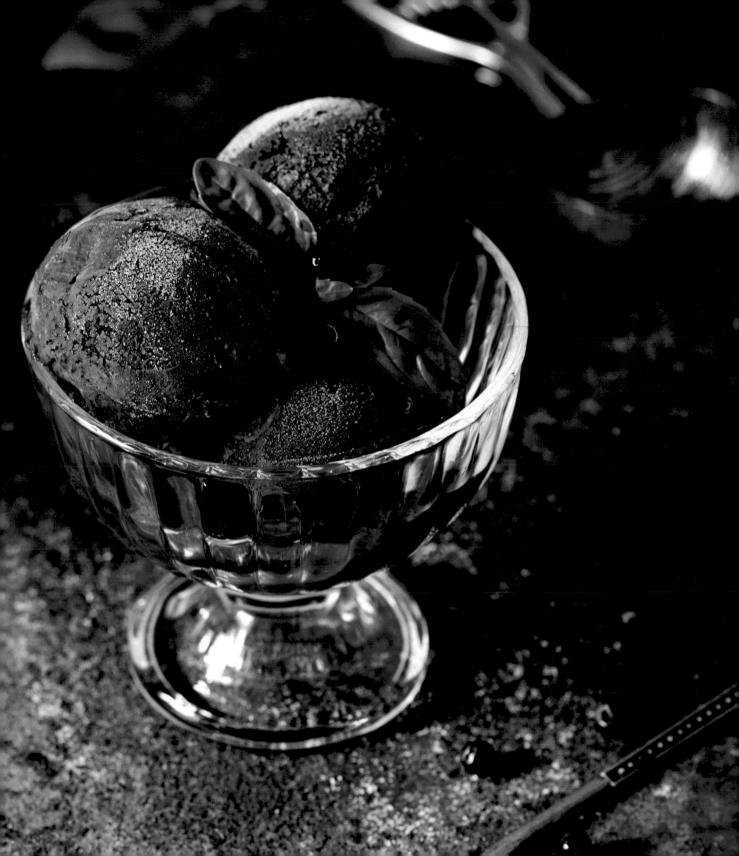

BLUEBERRY BASIL ICE CREAM

If you find yourself with an excess of blueberries come summer, you should freeze them.
You'll have a nutritious ingredient you can add to your recipes all year long.

INGREDIENTS

DIRECTIONS

SERVES 8

- 4 cups frozen blueberries
- 2 tablespoons honey
- ¼ cup water
- 4 cups coconut cream*
- ¼ teaspoon vanilla bean caviar
- ⅛ teaspoon sea salt
- 2 tablespoons fresh basil, minced

*Refrigerate four cans of coconut cream overnight. Only use the hardened coconut cream; reserve the liquid for another use.

Place the blueberries, honey and water in a small saucepan over medium-high heat. Stirring often, cook until the fruit is soft and the water has almost evaporated. Set aside and let cool completely.

Stir together the blueberry mixture, coconut cream, vanilla, salt, and basil. Transfer to an ice-cream maker and follow the manufacturer's instructions. Place the ice cream into the freezer to freeze for at least 2 hours.

PER SERVING: Calories: 400, Fat: 34.5g, Protein: 4.4g, Sodium: 65.5mg, Fiber: 1.8g, Carbohydrates: 20g, Sugar: 16g

PAPAYA SHERBET

This refreshing dessert shines in its simplicity! If you'd like,
swap out the papayas for frozen berries or melons.

INGREDIENTS

DIRECTIONS

SERVES 2-4

- 6 cups papaya
- ¾ cup date sugar
- 1 cup water

Peel and deseed the papayas, cut into 1-inch chunks and freeze.

In a small saucepan over medium heat, add the sugar and water. Let the water come to a simmer and stir until the sugar dissolves. Turn off the heat and let the mixture cool.

Place the frozen papayas in a blender with the sugar and water mixture. Blend until smooth. Place in a container and transfer to the freezer until firm, about 1 to 3 hours.

PER SERVING: Calories: 180, Fat: 0.5g, Protein: 1g, Sodium: 17mg, Fiber: 3.6g, Carbohydrates: 45g, Sugar: 34g

CHOCOLATE BARK

This simple, delicious bark is ideal for when you need a chocolate fix before bed. Feel free to switch out the coconut and pistachios for your favorite flavors.

INGREDIENTS	DIRECTIONS	SERVES 12

INGREDIENTS

- 12 ounces dark chocolate, with 80% cocoa
- ¼ cup unsweetened shredded coconut
- ½ cup pistachios
- 1 tablespoon coarse pink Himalayan sea salt

DIRECTIONS

Make a double boiler by adding 1 to 2 inches of water to a small saucepan and placing a small heat-proof bowl on top, making sure the bowl does not touch the water. Bring the water to a simmer. Add in the chocolate and turn off the heat. Let the chocolate melt, stirring occasionally with a rubber spatula.

Line a sheet pan with foil or parchment paper. Pour the melted chocolate onto the pan and spread into an even layer. Sprinkle the coconut and pistachios evenly onto the melted chocolate. Let the chocolate cool a little and sprinkle the sea salt on. Let the chocolate harden. Break into desired-size pieces and serve.

PER SERVING: Calories: 189, Fat: 15g, Protein: 3.2g, Sodium: 457mg, Fiber: 3.4g, Carbohydrates: 15g, Sugar: 8.4g

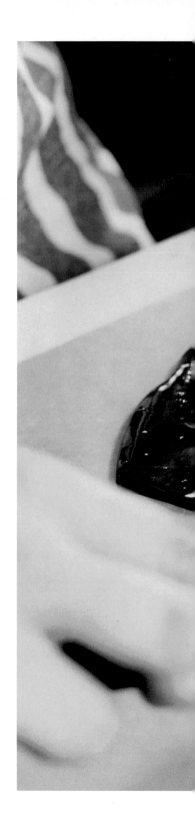

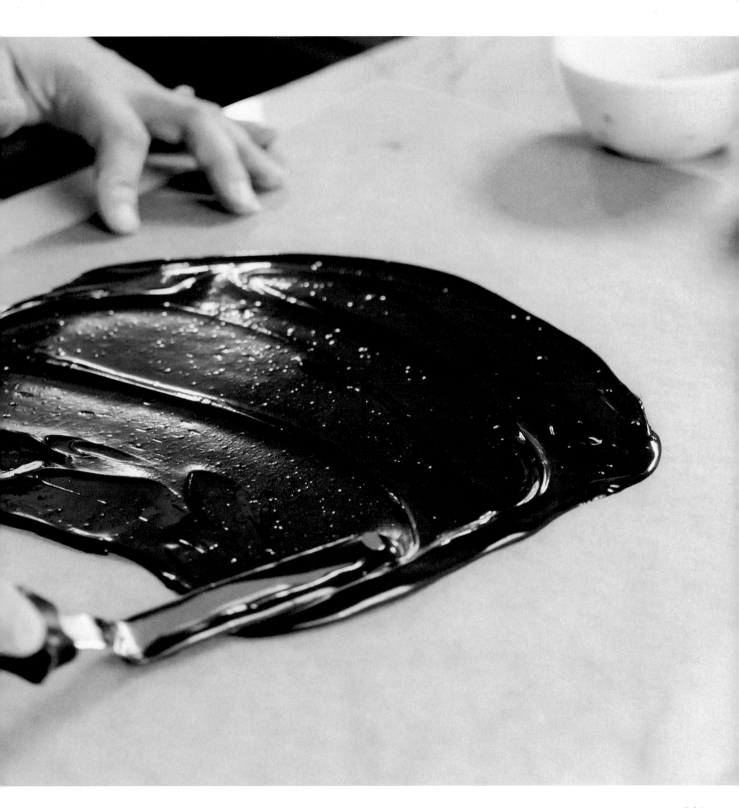

CHOCOLATE CHIP SKILLET BROWNIES

We all love a one-skillet dinner, but one-skillet desserts are even better. This pan is full of chocolatey, gooey deliciousness—it's everything you want from a brownie.

INGREDIENTS

DIRECTIONS

SERVES 8

- 1 tablespoon coconut oil
- 3 large eggs
- ½ cup honey
- 1 cup pumpkin purée
- 1 teaspoon vanilla bean caviar
- ½ cup coconut flour
- ½ cup unsweetened dark cocoa powder
- ¼ cup coconut sugar
- 1 teaspoon instant coffee
- 1 teaspoon baking powder
- ⅓ cup mini dark chocolate chips
- ½ cup chopped nuts (optional)

Preheat oven to 350 degrees F.

Grease a 10-inch cast-iron skillet with coconut oil.

In a large bowl, mix together the eggs, honey, pumpkin and vanilla until smooth. Add the flour, cocoa powder, sugar, instant coffee, baking powder, chocolate chips and chopped nuts, if using. Stir until combined.

Pour the batter into the greased skillet and place in the preheated oven. Bake for 40 minutes. Let cool slightly before slicing.

PER SERVING: Calories: 250, Fat: 11g, Protein: 5.5g, Sodium: 121mg, Fiber: 6.1g, Carbohydrates: 79g, Sugar: 28g

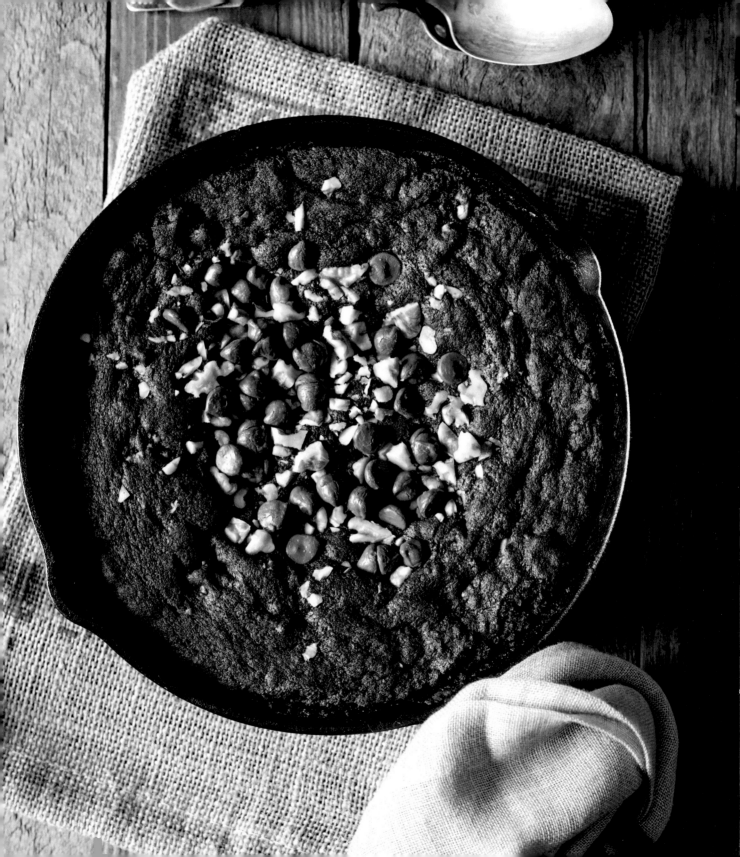

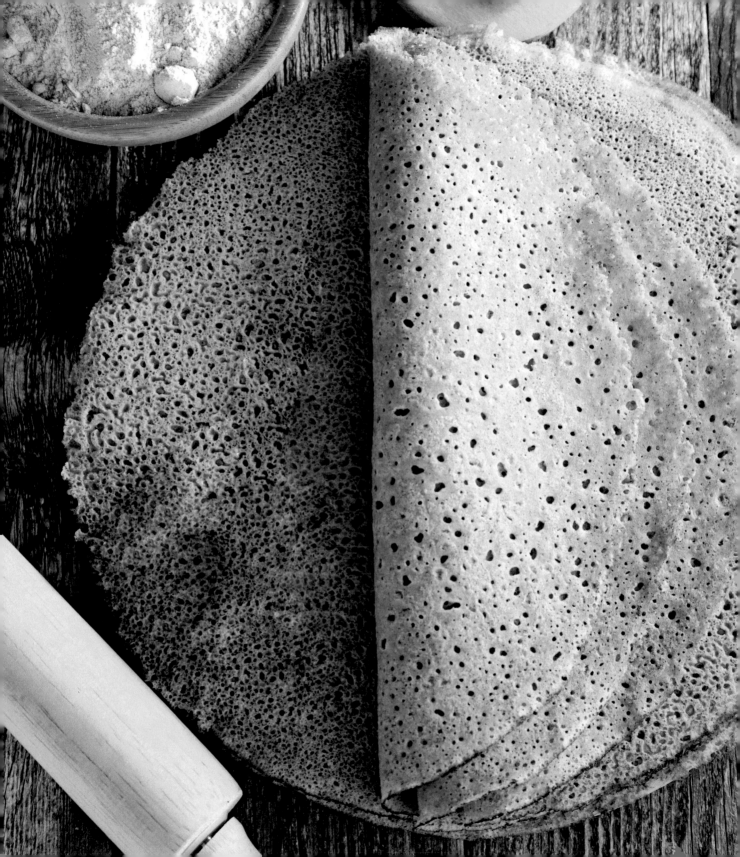

PUDDING-FILLED CREPE CAKE WITH BERRIES

This crepe cake uses the Peppery Pudding (page 197), which doubles as a frosting. The crushed pink peppercorns on top of the berries are optional, but we don't suggest skipping them.

INGREDIENTS   DIRECTIONS   SERVES 8

CAKE

- 1 cup millet flour
- 1 cup brown rice flour
- 2½ cups unsweetened almond milk
- 2 avocados
- 2 tablespoons maple syrup
- Pinch fine sea salt
- Ghee or butter for greasing pan
- Peppery Pudding (page 197)

TOPPINGS

- 2 cups mixed blueberries, blackberries and raspberries
- Crushed pink peppercorns, for garnish

In a blender, combine all cake ingredients except for the ghee and pudding. Blend until smooth.

Refrigerate the batter for 30 minutes.

In a nonstick pan over medium heat, add a thin coat of ghee and then place a thin coating (about ¼ cup) of batter into the pan, swirling to coat the pan evenly. Cook for about 1 minute, or until the batter starts to bubble, then flip and cook another minute. Remove from the pan and set aside. Continue in the same manner, greasing the pan for each crepe, until batter is gone. Place parchment paper between the crepes.

Cut the crepes to perfectly fit inside a springform pan. Place a crepe on the bottom of the pan, then place a thin layer of pudding on top of the crepe, evenly spreading it all the way to the edge. Continue layering until all of the ingredients are gone, saving some pudding for a slightly thicker layer at the top. Set the cake in the refrigerator to set for at least 2 hours.

Remove the cake from the springform pan and set on a cake plate or pedestal. Top with the remaining pudding, berries and crushed pink peppercorns.

PER SERVING: Calories: 489, Fat: 26.5g, Protein: 10.5g, Sodium: 127mg, Fiber: 18.5g, Carbohydrates: 62.5g, Sugar: 18g

STRAWBERRY CHEESECAKE

This classic strawberry cheesecake is light, fluffy and completely irresistible.
Don't be afraid to make it your own by using your favorite fruits.

INGREDIENTS | DIRECTIONS | SERVES 8

CRUST

1¼ cups almonds,
   crushed

¼ cup honey

FILLING

1 cup strawberries, plus
  extra for top if desired

1 tablespoon coconut
  sugar

⅔ cup full-fat coconut
  milk, refrigerated
  overnight

½ cup raw cashews,
  quick-soaked*

1 tablespoon fresh
  lemon juice

⅓ cup coconut oil,
  melted

½ cup honey

1 teaspoon vanilla bean
  caviar

*To quick-soak cashews,
pour boiling-hot water
over the cashews, soak
for 1 hour uncovered,
then drain and use as
instructed.

In a food processor, pulse the nuts and honey until a chunky paste forms. Press the mixture into the bottom and slightly up the sides of a springform pan.

In a small saucepan over medium heat, add the strawberries, sugar and ¼ cup water. Cook the strawberries until soft. Strain the mixture through a mesh colander.

Spoon ⅔ cup hardened coconut milk into a blender. Add the cashews, lemon juice, coconut oil, honey and vanilla. Blend together until smooth. Pour the mixture into the crust and swirl in the strawberry mixture, taking care to not disturb the crust. Place in the freezer for 3 to 4 hours. Once frozen, remove from the springform pan and garnish with fresh strawberries, if desired.

PER SERVING: Calories: 403, Fat: 28g, Protein: 6.8g, Sodium: 9.8mg,
Fiber: 3.4g, Carbohydrates: 38g, Sugar: 29g

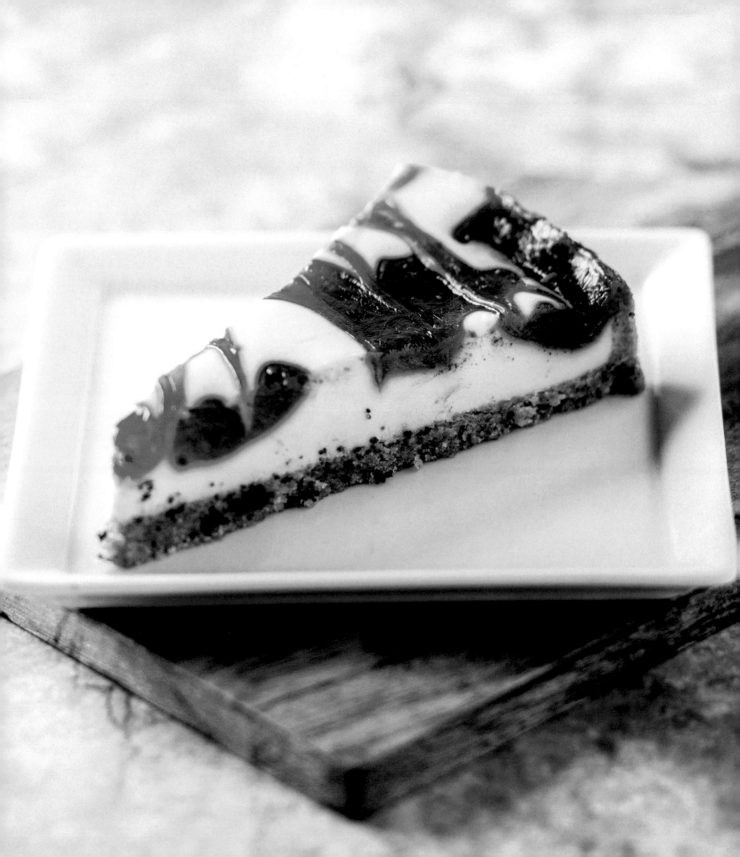

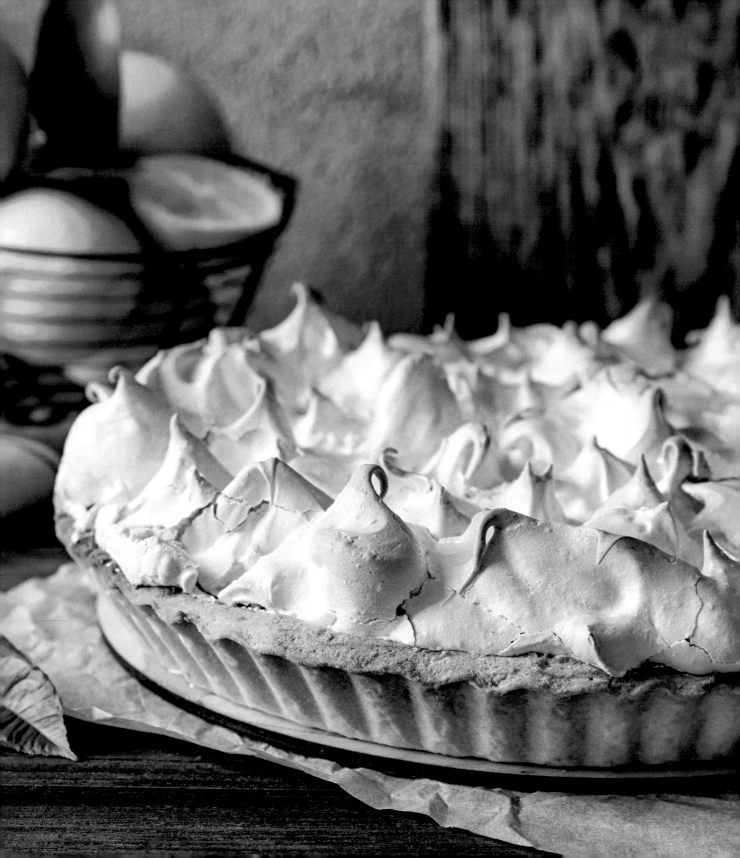

LEMON MERINGUE PIE

Lemon meringue pie is a must-have dessert! This classic has been brought back in a new, pegan-friendly way.

INGREDIENTS

CRUST

- 1½ cups almond flour
- 2 tablespoons coconut sugar
- ¼ teaspoon salt
- ¼ cup butter, melted

FILLING

- 2 (13.5-ounce) cans full-fat coconut milk
- ½ cup raw honey
- ½ cup fresh lemon juice, plus zest of 1 lemon
- 3 egg yolks, whites reserved for meringue

MERINGUE

- 3 egg whites, room temperature
- ¼ teaspoon cream of tartar
- 5 tablespoons coconut sugar
- ½ teaspoon vanilla bean caviar

DIRECTIONS

SERVES 8

Preheat oven to 325 degrees F.

Mix together all pie crust ingredients in a medium bowl. Press the mixture into the bottom and up the sides of a pie plate. Pierce the bottom crust with a fork. Place in the oven and cook for 10 minutes. Remove from the oven and let cool completely on a wire rack.

In a medium saucepan over medium-low heat, bring the coconut milk to a gentle simmer, then whisk in the honey. Simmer (do not let the mixture boil) over medium-low heat, about 30 to 40 minutes, until slightly thickened and reduced by ⅓. Take off the heat and cool. Measure 14 ounces for this recipe and reserve the rest (use it as you would sweetened condensed milk).

Raise the temperature of the oven to 350 degrees F.

In a medium bowl, whisk together the condensed milk, lemon juice, lemon zest and egg yolks. Pour the mixture into the crust and bake for 15 minutes. Cover the crust with foil if it gets too brown. Remove from the oven and let cool on a wire rack. Place in the refrigerator until chilled, preferably overnight.

Beat the egg whites and cream of tartar with an electric mixer on medium speed until foamy and soft peaks form. Change the speed to high and slowly add the sugar, mixing thoroughly after each addition. Continue beating until stiff peaks form and the sugar is completely dissolved. Beat in the vanilla.

Place the meringue on top of the pie to cover the filling. With the back of a spoon, lift the meringue to form peaks. Toast the peaks with a torch until the top is golden brown.

PER SERVING: Calories: 349, Fat: 26g, Protein: 7.6g, Sodium: 99mg, Fiber: 2.3g, Carbohydrates: 26g, Sugar: 20g

COCONUT, MATCHA AND KIWI PARFAIT

Matcha is a green tea filled with amazing amounts of antioxidants, making it an excellent ingredient for adding a nutritious boost to this tropical dessert.

INGREDIENTS

- 8 kiwis
- 1 cup coconut cream
- 1 tablespoon honey
- Juice of ½ lime
- 1 teaspoon matcha green tea powder
- Zest of 1 lime
- ½ cup shaved coconut, toasted
- 4 sprigs mint

DIRECTIONS

Peel the kiwis. Using a small melon baller, make kiwi balls from the kiwis.

In a small bowl, whisk together the coconut cream, honey, juice of ½ lime and matcha green tea powder.

Evenly fill four serving glasses with the coconut cream mixture. Top with the kiwi balls and garnish each with the lime zest, shaved coconut and a sprig of mint.

PER SERVING: Calories: 336, Fat: 23g, Protein: 4.9g, Sodium: 14mg, Fiber: 5.8g, Carbohydrates: 34g, Sugar: 23g

SERVES 4

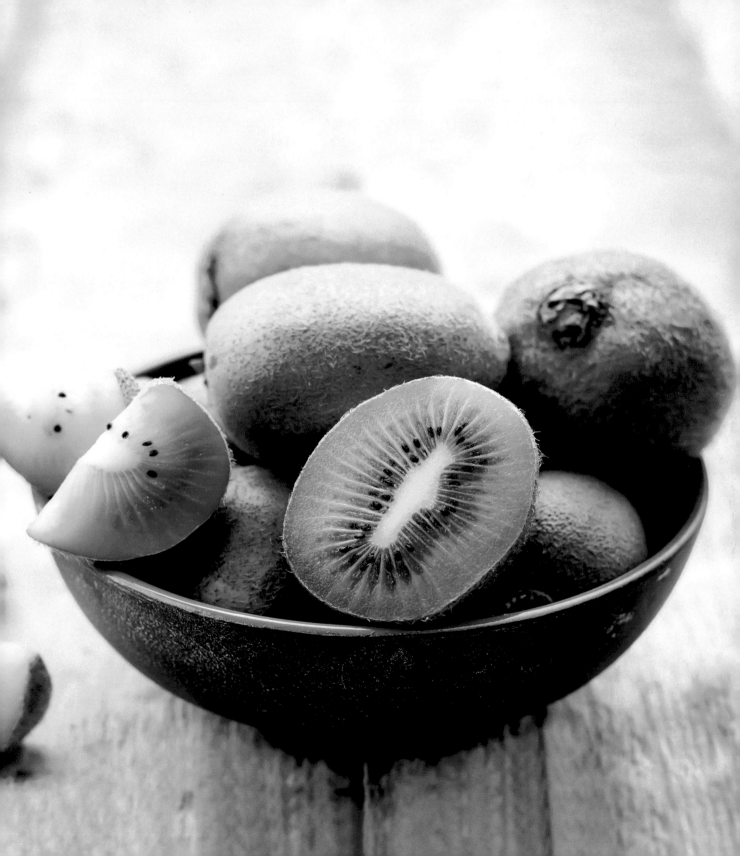

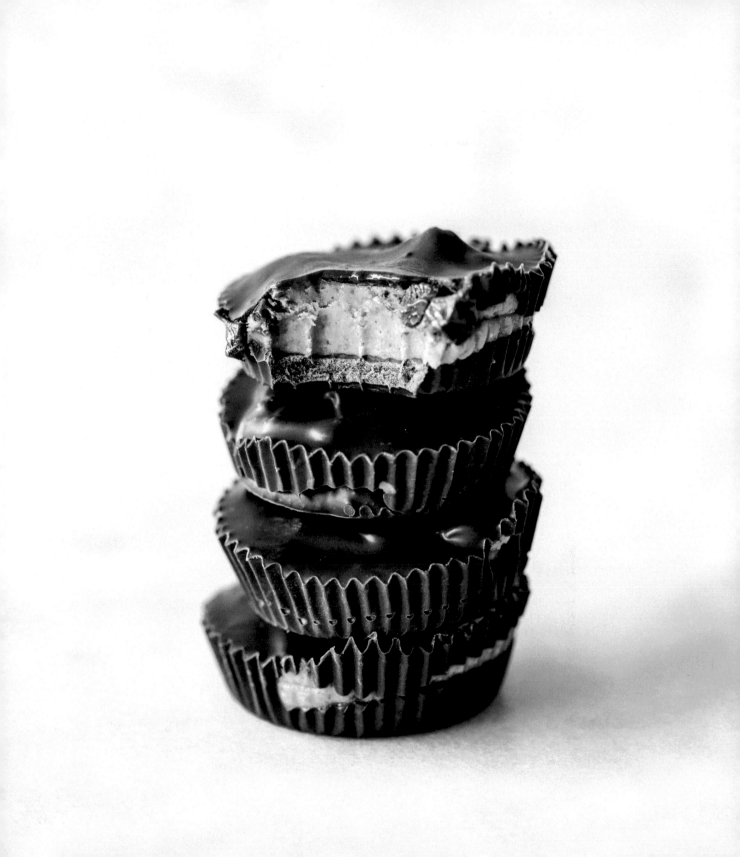

PEANUT BUTTER CUPS

Skip the extra sugar and preservatives by making your own peanut butter cups!
And don't be afraid to get creative—use any filling you'd like in these easy candies.

INGREDIENTS

- 8 ounces dark chocolate
- ½ cup natural peanut butter

DIRECTIONS

Make a double boiler by adding 1 to 2 inches of water to a small saucepan and placing a small heat-proof bowl on top, making sure the bowl does not touch the water. Bring the water to a simmer. Add the chocolate and turn off the heat. Let the chocolate melt, stirring occasionally with a rubber spatula.

Fill mini cupcake wrappers with 1 tablespoon chocolate, then place a teaspoon dollop of peanut butter in each. Place in the refrigerator to cool. Once cooled, top with another tablespoon melted chocolate and place in the refrigerator to set.

PER SERVING: Calories: 210, Fat: 16g, Protein: 5.3g, Sodium: 29mg, Fiber: 3.5g, Carbohydrates: 13g, Sugar: 7.3g

MERINGUE COOKIES

Don't be too intimidated by meringues—they're very simple, though they do take some time. Plan on baking these treats the day before you want to serve them.

INGREDIENTS

- 3 large egg whites, room temperature
- ⅛ teaspoon cream of tartar
- Pinch sea salt
- ¾ cup coconut sugar
- ½ teaspoon vanilla bean caviar

DIRECTIONS   MAKES 45 COOKIES

Preheat oven to 250 degrees F.

Line two sheet pans with parchment.

With an electric mixer fitted with a whisk attachment, whisk the egg whites on medium until light and airy and soft peaks form. Add the cream of tartar and salt. Increase the mixing speed to high and slowly add in the sugar and vanilla, beating after each addition until hard peaks form.

Place the mixture into a piping bag. (Use a decorative tip, if you'd like.) Pipe uniform 1½-inch dollops onto the parchment, spacing 1 inch apart.

Bake in the oven for 1 hour. Turn off the heat and let the cookies stay in the oven for at least 3 hours or overnight.

PER SERVING: Calories: 13, Fat: 0g, Protein: 0.2g, Sodium: 11mg, Fiber: 0g, Carbohydrates: 3.2g, Sugar: 3.2g

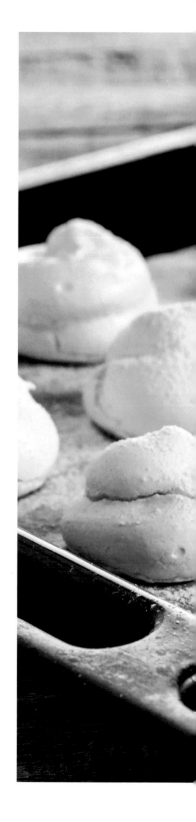

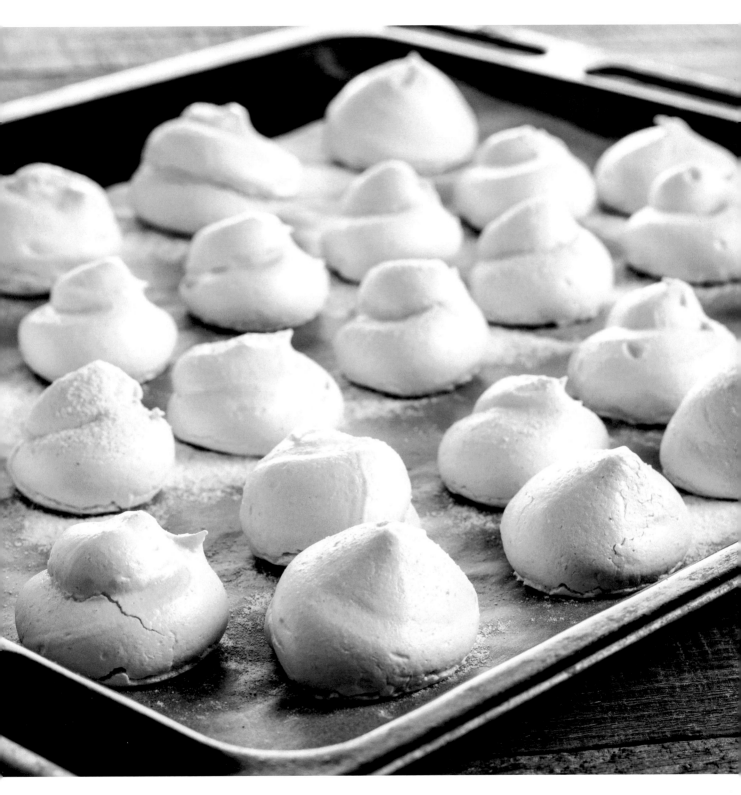

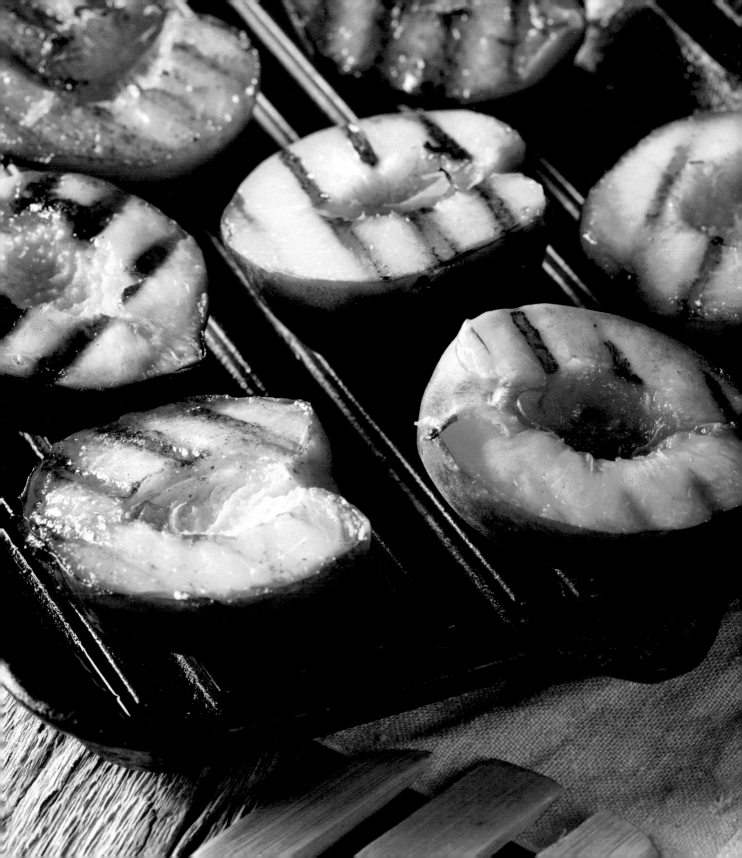

GRILLED NECTARINES

Grilling fruit caramelizes the sugars, making a naturally sweet and healthy dessert.

INGREDIENTS

- 4 large nectarines
- 1 tablespoon coconut oil
- 1½ cups coconut cream
- 1 tablespoon coconut sugar
- 1½ cups shaved coconut, toasted

DIRECTIONS

SERVES 6-8

Slice the nectarines in half and remove the pits. Brush each nectarine with coconut oil.

In a small bowl, mix together the coconut cream and coconut sugar.

Grill the nectarines on a hot grill until grill marks are achieved and the nectarines are slightly softened.

Place the nectarine halves in a serving bowl or plate. Top each with an even amount of coconut cream mixture and top with toasted coconut.

PER SERVING: Calories: 333, Fat: 29g, Protein: 3.8g, Sodium: 16mg, Fiber: 4g, Carbohydrates: 17g, Sugar: 12g

PUMPKIN PIE PARFAIT

This lighter version of pumpkin pie is a scrumptious way to end a fall meal.

| INGREDIENTS | DIRECTIONS | SERVES 8 |

INGREDIENTS

PUMPKIN PIE FILLING

- 2 cups pumpkin purée (not pumpkin pie filling)
- 1 can coconut cream, chilled overnight
- 3 tablespoons coconut sugar
- 1 teaspoon cinnamon
- ½ teaspoon nutmeg
- ½ teaspoon ground ginger
- ½ teaspoon vanilla extract
- ½ teaspoon sea salt

WHIPPED CREAM

- 2 cans coconut cream, chilled overnight
- ⅛ teaspoon cream of tartar
- 4 tablespoons coconut sugar

TOPPINGS (OPTIONAL)

- 2 cups pecans, chopped
- ¼ cup honey

DIRECTIONS

After chilling the coconut cream, half of the can will be liquid and the other half will be a thick layer of hardened coconut cream. In a blender, blend the pumpkin purée, hardened coconut cream, sugar, cinnamon, nutmeg, ginger, vanilla and sea salt until smooth.

For the whipped cream, use the hardened coconut cream from the remaining two cans and place in the bowl of a stand mixer. On medium speed, beat the coconut cream with the cream of tartar. When the coconut cream begins to whip up and become light and fluffy, turn the mixer on high and slowly add in the sugar. Continue to beat until silky and hard peaks form.

In four parfait glasses, place an even layer each of the pumpkin pie filling, whipped cream, nuts and a drizzle of honey. Continue to layer in the same way until all ingredients are used and the glasses are full. Top each with whipped cream and serve.

PER SERVING: Calories: 537, Fat: 45.5g, Protein: 6g, Sodium: 114mg, Fiber: 4.9g, Carbohydrates: 32g, Sugar: 25g

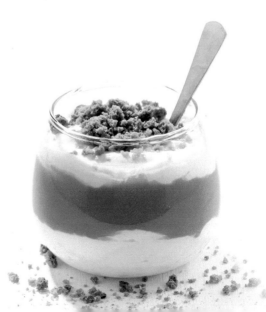

references

Adams, Shahieda, Andreas L. Lopata, Cornelius M. Smuts, Roslynn Baatjies, and Mohamed F. Jeebhay. "Relationship between Serum Omega-3 Fatty Acid and Asthma Endpoints." *International Journal of Environmental Research and Public Health* 16, no. 1 (January 2019): 43.

American Academy of Neurology. "Orange juice, leafy greens and berries may be tied to decreased memory loss in men." ScienceDaily, November 21, 2018. www.sciencedaily.com/releases/2018/11/181121171835.htm

American Thoracic Society. "Studies Find Eating Fruits and Vegetables Good for Lungs." ScienceDaily, May 22, 2001. www.sciencedaily.com/releases/2001/05/010522073859.htm

European Association for the Study of Obesity. "Eating a diet rich in fruit and vegetables could cut obesity risk." ScienceDaily, May 18, 2017. www.sciencedaily.com/releases/2017/05/170518220955.htm

Holt, Erica M., Lyn M. Steffen, Antoinette Moran, et al. "Fruit and vegetable consumption and its relation to markers of inflammation and oxidative stress in adolescents." *Journal of the Academy of Nutrition and Dietetics* 109, no. 3 (March 2009): 414–421.

Hyman, Mark. *Food: What the Heck Should I Eat?* New York: Little, Brown Spark, 2018.

Hyman, Mark. "This Weird Diet Is Actually the Healthiest, According to One of the Country's Top Functional Docs." mindbodygreen. www.mindbodygreen.com/articles/what-is-the-pegan-diet

Hyman, Mark. "Why I Am a Pegan—or Paleo-Vegan—and Why You Should Be Too!" (blog). November 7, 2014. Accessed July 11, 2019. drhyman.com/blog/2014/11/07/pegan-paleo-vegan

Lu, Yan, Ren-gang Chen, San-zou Wei, Han-guo Hu, Fei Sun, and Chun-hui Yu. "Effect of omega 3 fatty acids on C-reactive protein and interleukin-6 in patients with advanced nonsmall cell lung cancer." *Medicine* 97 (37): e11971 (September 2018).

Mayo Clinic. "DASH diet: Healthy eating to lower your blood pressure." www.mayoclinic.org/healthy-lifestyle/nutrition-and-healthy-eating/in-depth/dash-diet/art-20048456

National Institutes of Health. "Vitamin B12 Fact Sheet for Consumers." ods.od.nih.gov/factsheets/vitaminb12-healthprofessional

National Institutes of Health. "Vitamin D Fact Sheet for Health Professionals." ods.od.nih.gov/factsheets/VitaminD-HealthProfessional

Norwegian University of Science and Technology. "Eight servings of veggies a day is clearly best for the heart." ScienceDaily, February 23, 2017. www.sciencedaily.com/releases/2017/02/170223114807.htm

Rink, Stephanie M., Pauline Mendola, Sunni L. Mumford, et al. "Self-Report of Fruit and Vegetable Intake that Meets the 5 a Day Recommendation Is Associated with Reduced Levels of Oxidative Stress Biomarkers and Increased Levels of Antioxidant Defense in Premenopausal Women." *Journal of the Academy of Nutrition and Dietetics* 113, no. 6 (June 2013): 776–785.

University of Leeds. "Fruit and vegetables may be important for mental as well as physical well-being." ScienceDaily, February 5, 2019. www.sciencedaily.com/releases/2019/02/190205144450.htm

University of Southern California, Health Sciences. "Fruits and vegetables' latest superpower? Lowering blood pressure." ScienceDaily, April 5, 2017. www.sciencedaily.com/releases/2017/04/170405130950.htm

University of Warwick. "Fruit and veggies give you the feel-good factor." ScienceDaily, July 10, 2016. www.sciencedaily.com/releases/2016/07/160710094239.htm

index

A

Almond(s), 40, 56, 140, 193, 206
    butter, 40, 89
    flour, 162, 191, 192, 209
    milk, 40, 51, 59, 60, 145,
        155, 169, 205
Anchovies, 93, 104, 154, 174
Apples, 102, 109
    honeycrisp, 89, 107, 132, 193
Arrowroot, 169
Artichokes, 91
Arugula, 101, 115
Asparagus, 83, 126, 141
Avocado(s), 37, 43, 44, 47, 51,
        60, 76, 82, 87, 98, 159,
        163, 182, 197, 205
    crema, 163
    oil, 82, 163

B

Baby bok choy, 130
Bacon, 39, 43, 59, 112
Baking powder, 48, 202
Beans
    black, 187
    red, 97
Beef
    baby back ribs, 181
    ground, 69, 172, 176, 184
    short ribs, bone-in, 153
    skirt steak, 83, 183

Beets, 63, 81, 99, 117, 126,
    133, 137
Berries, mixed, 48
Blackberries, 154, 191, 205
Blueberries, 40, 46, 63, 191, 205
    frozen, 199
Broccoli, 146, 183
Broth
    beef, 118, 153
    chicken, 110, 154, 158, 172,
        175, 179, 184
    vegetable, 55, 68, 97, 107, 110,
        115, 118, 129, 157, 160,
        167, 169, 170, 179, 187
Brussels sprouts, 69, 99, 102,
    136, 146

C

Cabbage, 132
    dark green, 166
    Napa, 99
    purple, red, 76, 91, 99
Capers, 158
Carrots, 55, 83, 90, 91, 97, 105,
    107, 115
Cauliflower, 39, 129, 140, 162,
    169
Celery, 55, 97, 107, 159
Cheese
    feta, 66
    goat, 39, 52, 59, 98, 133

Chicken, 90, 171
    breasts, 163
    cooked, 97, 110
    thighs, 175
    wings, 158
Chocolate
    chips, 56, 202
    dark, 200, 213
Clams, littleneck, 179
Cocoa powder, 197, 202
Coconut
    cream, 68, 193, 199, 210,
        217, 218
    flour, 73, 93, 202
    milk, 107, 197, 206, 209
    oil, 192, 202, 206, 217
    shaved, shredded, 47, 56,
        63, 73, 200, 210, 217
    sugar, 56, 191, 192, 193, 197,
        202, 206, 209, 214,
        217, 218
Coffee, 197, 202
Crabmeat, 51
Cucumber, 70, 98, 101, 108, 109,
    132

D

Dragon fruit, 197

E

Eggplant, 55, 70, 176

F

Flour
    almond, *see Almonds*
    brown rice, 51, 60, 205
    coconut, *see Coconut*
    millet, 51, 60, 205
Flowers, edible, 117

G

Ghee, 174, 205
Ginger, 105, 110, 115, 130, 134, 181, 183
Grapefruit, 104
Green beans, 126, 174
    Chinese long, 104

H

Herbs
    basil, 55, 66, 73, 98, 104, 108, 138, 157, 170, 175, 176, 182, 199
    chives, 43, 54, 59, 68, 81, 90, 145, 159
    cilantro, 76, 87, 115, 141, 163
    dill, 70, 109, 132
    mint, 47, 48, 60, 210
    oregano, 104, 126
    parsley, 55, 68, 73, 78, 84, 90, 98, 104, 110, 126, 129, 132, 142, 153, 157, 158, 160, 166, 167, 169, 170, 174, 176, 179

rosemary, 153, 157, 165, 175, 187
sage, 107
thyme, 70, 83, 104, 118, 153, 154, 167, 175, 187
Honey, 40, 47, 56, 105, 117, 130, 134, 148, 160, 172, 183, 186, 191, 192, 193, 194, 199, 202, 206, 209, 210, 218
Horseradish, 73, 117, 137, 145, 158, 166

J

Juice
    lemon, 51, 63, 99, 102, 108, 109, 110, 117, 132, 147, 155, 158, 159, 174, 179, 191, 192, 193, 205, 209
    lime, 47, 62, 76, 87, 101, 115, 134, 141, 163, 210
    orange, 104, 181, 194

K

Kale, 55, 63, 75, 91, 99, 105
Ketchup, Pegan, 73, 160, 172
Kiwi, 47, 210
Kombucha, 63

L

Lamb chops, 154
Leeks, 68, 142, 146, 165, 169

Lemon(s), 70, 91, 121, 130
    juice, *see Juice*
    zest, 48, 70, 93, 99, 109, 110, 126, 158, 174, 179, 209
Lentils, 81
Lettuce
    romaine, 81, 108, 182
    butter, 99, 162, 165
    frisée, 104
    bib, 159
    artisan mix, 182
Lime(s)
    juice, *see Juice*
    zest, 47, 141, 171, 210

M

Maple syrup, 39, 51, 60, 205
Matcha green tea powder, 47, 63, 210
Microgreens, 82, 174
Millet, uncooked, 40, 157
    flour, *see Flour*
Mushrooms
    cremini, 52, 170, 178, 184
    oyster, 142
    shiitake, 118, 167
Mussels, 160
Mustard, 121, 160, 184
    Dijon, 102
    whole grain, 112

N

Nectarines, 217
Noodles, soba, 134, 179
Nuts, 202
    almonds, *see Almonds*
    cashews, 155, 205
    hazelnuts, 115
    macadamia, 56
    pecans, 89, 191, 218
    pine, 137, 166
    pistachios, 39, 56, 102, 140,
        182, 200
    walnuts, 56, 104, 192

O

Olives, Kalamata, 170
Onion(s), 43, 55, 59, 62, 69, 81,
    84, 90, 97, 107, 110, 138,
    172, 175, 176
    green, 73, 101, 171, 178, 179
    red, 76, 87, 98, 105, 109,
        132, 136, 170, 171
    sweet, 73, 187
Oranges, 60, 104, 181
    blood, 105, 194
    juice, *see Juice*
Oysters, 78

P

Papaya, 199
Pea shoots, 117, 182

Peaches, 66
Peanut butter, 213
Pears, 112, 194
Pepper(s), 59
    green, 175
    hot chili, 73, 108
    jalapeño, 76, 81, 87, 101, 132
    orange, 87, 166
    poblano, 163
    red, 43, 59, 62, 81, 83, 90,
        136, 137, 169, 170, 187
    yellow, 91
Pineapple, 171
Plums, 108, 186
Pomegranate, 60
    seeds, *see Seeds*
Pork
    butt, 172
    tenderloin, 186
Potatoes, fingerling, 43, 178
Prawns, 107
Prosciutto, 37, 44
Protein powder, vanilla-flavored
    vegan, 48
Pumpkin purée, 202, 218

Q

Quinoa, 44, 121, 165
    flakes, 192

R

Radicchio, 112
Radishes, 125
Raspberries, 46, 115, 191, 192,
    205
Rice
    black, 68, 136, 197
    red, 129

S

Salmon, 54, 70, 159, 160, 169
Salsa, 43, 81
Sardine fillets, 91
Sauce
    hot, 97, 160, 162
    marinara, 90, 176
    soy, 134, 160, 181, 183
Sausage link, 52
Scallops, 68, 174
Seeds
    chia, 40, 63, 176
    coriander, 140
    cumin, 140
    flaxseed, 108, 192
    hemp, 40
    pepitas, 115, 134
    pomegranate, 63, 102, 105
    poppy, 99
    sesame, 117, 134, 140, 183
Shallots, 102, 104, 112, 115, 129,
    154, 167, 178

Shrimp, 73, 87, 170, 178
Spices
    basil, 74, 184
    blackened seasoning, 178
    Cajun seasoning, 107
    cayenne pepper, 78, 115,
        134, 171, 182
    celery seed, 132
    chili powder, 62, 140, 172,
        187
    chipotle powder, 141, 163
    cinnamon, 40, 89, 191, 192,
        193, 194, 197, 218
    cream of tartar, 193, 209,
        214, 218
    cumin, 81, 163, 187
    dukkah, 75, 82, 140
    five-spice, 115, 134
    garlic powder, 74, 162, 163
    ginger, 182, 218
    hamburger seasoning, 69
    Italian seasoning, 90
    mustard powder, 163
    nutmeg, 107, 218
    onion powder, 74, 155, 162
    oregano, 74, 163
    paprika, 171
    parsley, 74, 171, 184
    pumpkin spice, 107

    red pepper flakes, 70, 93,
        142, 165, 174, 181
    rosemary, 186
    thyme, 186
    turmeric, 115, 182
Spinach, 52, 55, 90, 169
    baby, 54, 78, 118, 172
Squash, 55, 90
    butternut, 107, 134, 155
    Kabocha, 147
    spaghetti, 84
Strawberries, 46, 191, 206
Sweet potatoes, 62, 82, 89, 165,
    187
Swiss chard, 148

T
Tahini, 147, 181
Tomato(es), 47, 55, 68, 73, 74,
        76, 87, 170, 176
    cherry, 108, 138, 171
    crushed, canned, 175
    grape, 43, 54, 74, 98, 138, 174
    heirloom, 182
    paste, 129, 163
    plum, canned, 187
    sun-dried, 59
    vine, 44
Turmeric, fresh, 169
Turnip, 145

V
Vanilla, bean caviar, 40, 191,
        192, 194, 197, 199, 202,
        206, 209, 214, 218
Vegetable spread, 39, 55, 82
Vinegar
    apple cider, 101, 102, 109,
        112, 115, 130, 132, 163
    balsamic, 66, 73, 83, 99,
        105, 108, 125
    champagne, 117
    red wine, 98
    rice wine, 147
    sherry, 148
    white wine, 104, 121

Y
Yeast, 155
Yogurt, sheep's, 46, 47, 70, 97,
        107, 109, 115, 184

Z
Zucchini, 74, 138, 170, 178

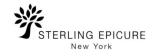

STERLING EPICURE
New York

An Imprint of Sterling Publishing Co., Inc.
1166 Avenue of the Americas
New York, NY 10036

ISBN 978-1-4549-3790-6

Distributed in Canada by Sterling Publishing Co., Inc.
c/o Canadian Manda Group, 664 Annette Street
Toronto, Ontario M6S 2C8, Canada
Distributed in the United Kingdom by GMC Distribution Services
Castle Place, 166 High Street, Lewes, East Sussex BN7 1XU, England
Distributed in Australia by NewSouth Books
University of New South Wales, Sydney, NSW 2052, Australia

For information about custom editions, special sales, and premium and corporate purchases, please
contact Sterling Special Sales at 800-805-5489 or specialsales@sterlingpublishing.com.

Manufactured in China

2 4 6 8 10 9 7 5 3 1

sterlingpublishing.com

Recipes by Isabel Minunni
Text and nutritional data by Aimee McNew, MNT, CNTP
Cover design by David Ter-Avanesyan
Indexing by R studio T, NYC

Photo Credits:
iStock/Getty Images: arfo: 185; bohofack2: back cover; knape: 17; letterberry: 196; Qwart: 215; Dmitry_Tsvetkov: 13
Shutterstock: 135pixels: 180; Africa Studio: 208; Nataliya Arzamasova: 211; AS Food Studio: 128, 177, 216; baibaz: 32; bergamont: 171; Binh Thanh Bui: 54; Rimma Bondarenko: 7; Tatiana Bralnina: 49; Natasha Breen: back cover, 61, 131; caldix: 141; j.chizhe: 57; Steve Cukrov: 143; Da-ga: 137; DronG: 79; Barbara Dudzinska: 34, 45; Amallia Eka: 135; Andrey Eremin: 105; Slawomir Fajer: 53; Nina Firsova: 75; from my point of view: 106, 156; gresei: 162; HandmadePictures: 127; Alexis Harrison: front cover; Brent Hofacker: back cover, 72, 80, 86, 88; Oliver Hoffmann: 192; Jiang Hongyan: 159; ifong: 46; Jaycee3663: 116; Tomo Jesenicnik: 9; jultud: 36; KarepaStock: 173; Emily Li: 146, 167; Bartosz Luczak: 42; Jacob Lund: 19; margouillat photo: 204; msheldrake: 182; Lapina Maria: 100; Olga Miltsova: 108; Anastasiia Moses: 212; MRAORAOR: 98; MShev: 58; Lisovskaya Natalia: 144, 161; New Africa: 120; Vladislav Noseek: 149; PIXbank CZ: 69; Andrey_Popov: 23; Anna_Pustynnikova: 96; Rawpixel.com: 5; RelentlessImages: 207; Irina Rostokina: 64, 77, 114; Artem Samokhvalov: 63; ScenaStudio: 154; Sea Wave: 41; Elzbieta Sekowska: 111; Siim79: 164; Sokorevaphoto: back cover, 188, 198; SOMMAI: 82; Chatnarung Srangkusol: 132; StockphotoVideo: 94, 119; William Stubbs: 152; thefoodphotographer: 38, 103, 195; Tiger Images: 91, 175, 178, 187; Alex Tihonovs: 92; tmcphotos: 21; Ksenija Toyechkina: 71; Natalia Van Doninck: 50; VDB Photos: 190; Elena Veselova: 203; vm2002Y: 85; Natalia Wimberley: 219; Y Photo Studio: 67; zoryanchik: 124, 150, 168
Stocksy: Suzanne Clements: 30; Nadine Greeff: 26; Ina Peters: 122, 139; Pixel Stories: 113; Trinette Reed: 15; Martí Sans: 24; Good Vibrations Images: 11; Cameron Whitman: 201